Ketogenic Diet, My Spiralized Cookbook, Sugar Detox And Clean Eating Box Set:

Over 100 Delicious And Healthy Recipes For Weight Loss And Fat Burning

by Eric Deen

Published in United States by:

Eric Deen

© Copyright 2015 – Eric Deen

ISBN-13: 978-1518845253
ISBN-10: 1518845258

Table of Contents

Chapter 3:

Chapter 4:

Book 1
Ketogenic Diet for Beginners: 40+ Delicious Ketogenic Recipes for Weight loss & Fat Burning 7 Day Meal Planner Included!

Introduction

Ready to learn Delicious Ketogenic Recipes for Weight loss & Fat Burning?

You have made a step in the right direction by downloading this book. It shows that you truly want to begin living a healthier lifestyle that will result in weight loss and fat burning. This is a great diet choice especially for those that have type two diabetes or are concerned about developing diabetes and other life threatening medical conditions.

The ketogenic diet has been used as a form of treatment of epilepsy for many years. The ketogenic diet is meant to maintain the fasting metabolism over a long space of time. During this fasting state the body creates ketones, these are a by-product of the fat-burning metabolism. Individuals that have epilepsy have found that their seizures disappear or lessen during these fasting periods.

The ketogenic diet is low in carbohydrates and high in fats. Ketones become formed when the primary source of calories is coming from fat stored in our bodies. When the body is in ketosis it has higher than normal levels of ketones in the blood. In a ketogenic state the body's lipid energy metabolic is intact.

The main benefit of ketosis is that it helps to increase your body's ability to make use of stored fats for fuel, when the body is no longer getting high-carbohydrates it is forced then to become efficient in using fats as an energy source.

The second benefit to ketosis is that it has a protein-sparing effect, assuming that you are already consuming an adequate amount of calories per day. Once the body is in ketosis it prefers ketones to glucose.

The best place to start when making healthy changes in your life is finding a diet that is going to be beneficial to you and your health and well-being. In this fast paced world that we live in today it is vital that we make an effort to provide ourselves with a well-balanced diet that will enable us to function at our best. A healthy diet will help to ensure that our chances of developing certain diseases like heart disease will be greatly reduced. Providing your body with a healthy diet will allow it to operate on a healthy level that you in turn will feel more energized, feeling great as you lose those unwanted pounds!

To make the ketogenic diet work for you then you must be prepared to avoid cheating on this diet, make sure that you are eating what is needed in order for you to be satiated or full. You must remember that Ketosis is a process that happens in your body. This takes time and it takes sticking to the diet. If you go off the diet it could take your body another week to get back to the state of ketosis again. So before you begin this diet make sure that you are ready to be fully committed to it if not then it just won't work otherwise. Some people find setting a start date for new things in their life such as starting a diet or quitting smoking etc. This process can help you both mentally and physically prepare for the start date. By putting it into your personal calendar this makes the commitment seem more solid and real. I wish you the best of luck in finding your way to better health through the ketogenic diet. I hope the recipes and meal planner I have provided will help make your journey a little easier!

Chapter 1:
Beginning a Ketogenic Diet

If you have planned starting the diet with empty cupboards so that you will fill them with the foods that you will need for the ketogenic diet then your first week's shopping list may include some specialty items such as almond flour, Stevia, milled flaxseed meal, and coconut flour. You should be able to find Stevia (natural sweetener) at most grocery stores. The other specialty items you may have to take a run to your local health food store to pick up.

Week 1. In the first week of the ketogenic diet plan I want to keep it simple so that it will be an easy process for you in just starting out on a low carb diet. If you make it a difficult transition is will just become torturous when you are having those hard to get rid of cravings. In some of the recipes you will have leftovers that you can freeze and use at a later date which will save you from cooking one less meal—a bit of a time saver for you.

The first signs of ketosis are commonly referred to as "keto flu" where you may experience fatigue, brain fogginess, and headaches. It is very important that you make sure that you are drinking plenty of water and eating salt. You are going to find that during the ketogenic diet you will be peeing a lot more as it is a diuretic. Electrolytes are removed from the body during this time. It is important that you make sure that your intake of water and salt is at a level that will allow your body to re-hydrate and re-supply electrolytes. By making sure to do this you will avoid the headaches. You can sprinkle some salt into your water that you are drinking. You should drink four liters of water a day, and keep taking some salt as well. If you are worried about the salt intake affecting your high blood pressure, don't as there has been recent findings that sodium intake and blood pressure are not correlated as we once believed that they were.

Breakfast. I would suggest when you start your diet begin day one on a weekend, then you can make something that can last you for the entire week for breakfast. Nobody wants to be bothered making something before they have to rush out the door for work.

Lunch. For the first week of lunches keeping them simple is the best way. This is going to involve salad and meat that will be covered in some kind of yummy high fat dressing. Use meats from the dinner of the night before to make the next day lunch with. You can add spices to your salad, but be careful on the amounts of onion and garlic powders.

Dinner. Dinner is going to involve more veggies and meat, going high on the good fats and moderate on the protein. There is no desert for the first two weeks of the ketogenic diet plan.

Week One's Shopping List

Cheese:

- cheddar cheese (full fat)
- Queso Fresco Cheese or Paneer cheese
- Parmesan cheese

Vegetables:

- sugar snap peas
- lots of spinach
- parsley
- orange
- green beans
- cauliflower
- broccoli
- six lemons
- three yellow onions
- one green pepper

Spices:

- salt

- sage
- cardamom
- cayenne
- rosemary
- chili powder
- oregano
- coconut flour
- onion powder
- ginger
- cumin
- paprika
- red pepper flakes
- chives
- minced garlic
- black pepper
- allspice
- bay leaf
- yellow curry powder
- xanthan gum
- thyme

Sauces:

- Worcestershire
- fish sauce (gluten free)
- Tomato sauce (low-carb brand)
- Soy sauce
- red wine
- ranch dressing (full fat)
- Dijon mustard
- coconut milk
- chicken stock
- beef broth

Meats & Poultry:

- Shrimp
- ground beef
- stew meat
- pork rinds
- eggs
- chicken thighs
- Chorizo Sausage
- Chicken Sausage
- canned chicken

- bacon

Fats:

- pecans
- half and half heavy cream
- coconut oil
- unsalted and salted grass fed butter
- bottle of olive oil
- save fat from bacon that you cook

Now that you have gathered your groceries to begin the ketogenic diet you are ready to begin your new healthy lifestyle the next chapter will get you started with your meal planner recipes for meals will be in later chapters.

Chapter 2- Meal Planner

Day 1

Breakfast

Scrambled Eggs with Cheese (page 57)

Per Serving.

Calories: 453

Fats: 43g

Net Carbs: 1.2g

Protein: 19g

Lunch

Canned Chicken & Spinach Salad (page 63)

Per Serving.

Calories: 450

Fats: 44g

Net Carbs: 0.5g

Protein: 13.5g

Dinner

Bacon Burger & Red Pepper Salad (page 59)

Per Serving.

Calories: 641

Fats: 52.5g

Net Carbs: 4.7g

Protein: 37g

Day Totals.

Calories: 1544

Fats: 1395

Net Carbs: 6.4

Proteins: 69.5

Day 2

Breakfast

Frittata Muffins (two muffins) (page 61)

Per Serving.

Calories: 410

Fats: 32.3g

Net Carbs: 2.5g

Protein: 27.3g

Lunch

Leftover Bacon Burger & Spinach Salad

Per Serving.

Calories: 624

Fats: 63.9g

Net Carbs: 1.2g

Protein: 10.8g

Dinner

Sausage & Chicken Stir Fry (page 64)

Freeze leftovers for two more meals, add one quarter of a cup of shredded cheddar to meal not to leftovers.

Per Serving.

Calories: 541

Fats: 8.3g

Net Carbs: 8.3g

Protein: 42.7g

Day Totals.

Calories: 1575

Fats: 104.5

Net Carbs: 12.

Protein: 42.7

Day 3

Breakfast

Frittata Muffins (two muffins) (page 61)

Per Serving.

Calories: 410

Fats: 32.3g

Net Carbs: 2.5g

Protein: 27.3g

Lunch

Spinach Salad (page 66)

Per Serving.

Calories: 537

Fats: 57g

Net Carbs: 1g

Dinner

Orange & Cinnamon Beef Stew (page 67)

Per Serving.

Calories: 519

Fats: 35.6g

Net Carbs: 4.1g

Protein: 42.8g

Day Totals.

Calories: 1466

Fats: 124.9

Net Carbs: 7.6

Proteins: 70.1

Day 4

Breakfast

Scrambled Eggs with Cheese (page 57)

Per Serving.

Calories: 453

Fats: 43g

Net Carbs: 1.2g

Protein: 19g

Lunch

Leftover Orange & Cinnamon Stew (page 67)

Per Serving.

Calories: 519

Fats: 35.6g

Net Carbs: 4.1g

Protein: 42.8g

Dinner

Shrimp & Cauliflower Curry (page 69)

(Eat one sixth of recipe and freeze the rest as five portions)

Per Serving.

Calories: 451

Fats: 33.5g

Net Carbs: 5.6g

Protein: 27.4g

Day Totals.

Calories: 1423

Fats: 112.1

Net Carbs: 10.9

Proteins: 89.2

Day 5

Breakfast

Frittata Muffins (two muffins) (page 61)

Per Serving.

Calories: 410

Fats: 32.3g

Net Carbs: 2.5g

Protein: 27.3g

Lunch

Leftover Chicken & Sausage & Spinach Salad (pages 64 and 66)

Per Serving.

Calories: 742

Fats: 70.2g

Net Carbs: 4.7g

Protein: 20.8g

Dinner

Curry Chicken Thigh with Fried Queso Fresco (page 71)

Per Serving.

Calories: 657

Fats: 44.7g

Net Carbs: 0.6g

Protein: 40.3g

Day Totals.

Calories: 1809

Fats: 147.2

Net Carbs: 7.8

Protein: 88.4

Day 6

Breakfast

Scrambled Eggs with Cheese (page 57)

Per Serving:

Calories: 453

Fats: 43g

Net Carbs: 1.2g

Protein: 19g

Lunch

Leftover Curry Chicken & Spinach Salad (pages 71 and 66)

Per Serving:

Calories: 586

Fats: 58g

Net Carbs: 1g

Protein: 15g

Dinner

Chorizo & Cheddar Meatballs (Eat five meatballs and freeze the leftovers) (page 73)

Roasted Pecan Green Beans (Eat half a serving and leftovers as five portions) (page 74)

Per Serving.

Calories: 798

Fats: 63g

Net Carbs: 7.1g

Protein: 40.2g

Day Totals.

Calories: 1837

Fats: 164

Net Carbs: 9.3

Protein: 74.2

Day 7

Breakfast

Scrambled Eggs with Cheese (page 57)

Per Serving.

Calories: 553

Fats: 55g

Net Carbs: 1.2g

Protein: 19g

Lunch

Spinach Salad with Cream Cheese (page 75)

Per Serving.

Calories: 496

Fats: 51g

Net Carbs: 2g

Proteins: 5g

Dinner

Chili (Eat one quarter of the total recipe freeze leftovers for three more portions) (page 76)

Sugar Snap Peas (Eat one third of total recipe and save

leftovers for two portions) (page 78)

Per Serving.

Calories: 545

Fats: 31.1g

Net Carbs: 9.6g

Proteins: 53.1g

Day Totals.

Calories: 1594

Fats: 136.1g

Week 2

Congratulations on making it through the first week of the ketogenic diet, hopefully you found it fairly easy to keep track of your food intake. We are going to introduce bullet proof coffee into the menu. This coffee is made from a blend of coconut oil, grass-fed butter, and heavy cream. You may be thinking what kind of weird concoction is this? Believe me it may sound strange but it is going to add a lovely decadent richness to your morning coffee, that I am sure you will quickly learn to enjoy and look forward to.

If you are someone who is not a fan of coffee then try it in your tea. The bullet proof coffee is great at helping with fat loss. In this coffee you will be taking in medium-chain triglycerides or MCT's that have been shown to lead to greater loses in fat tissue, in both animals and humans. By eating these fats you are going to have more efficient energy usage, and along with better results in weight loss.

Medium chain fatty acids or MCFAs lead to an increase in energy expenditure, they are converted into ketones, which are absorbed differently by the body compared to other oils, giving us better overall energy. You can add spices or sweeteners to this.

With your lunches you can continue to add leftovers from the night before. Using leftover meats from the previous night's dinner along with a green salad with high fat dressings. Just remember to balance out your proteins with your fats this is important.

Your dinner will still be fairly simple with meats, vegetables, along with the high fat dressings. You might wish to put some butter on your veggies at dinner. Just keep in mind that this simple menu spells success for you in reaching your goals of weight loss in a healthy manner, through the use of a healthy diet plan. There is to be no deserts in the second week of the diet plan either.

Shopping List for week 2
Specialty Items:

- milled flax seed
- almond flour

These items you will most likely have to go to your local health food store to purchase

Crunchy Items:

- pork rinds
- pecans
- almonds

Spices:

- Chipotle seasoning
- Mrs. Dash table blend
- baking soda
- baking powder

Vegetables:

- sugar snap peas

- spring onion
- mushrooms
- lemons
- green beans

Cheese:

- cheddar cheese
- mozzarella cheese
- cream cheese
- blue cheese crumbled

Sauces/Liquids

- yellow mustard
- hot sauce
- coffee
- apple cider vinegar

Meat:

- Chorizo Sausage
- chicken breast

Day 8

Breakfast

Bulletproof Coffee

Per Serving:

Calories: 273

Fats: 30g

Net Carbs: 1g

Protein: 0g

Lunch

Taco Tartlets (eat two for one serving)

Per Serving:

Calories: 481

Fats: 38.8g

Net Carbs: 5.47g

Protein: 26.2g

Dinner

Leftover Chorizo Meatballs (eat eight for dinner) along with one portion of Roasted Pecan Green Beans) (page 73)

Per Serving.

Calories: 921

Fats: 72.2 g

Net Carbs: 7.9g

Protein: 47.5g

Day Totals.

Calorie: 1675

Fats: 141

Net Carbs: 14.3

Proteins: 73.7

Day 9

Breakfast

Bulletproof Coffee

Per Serving:

Calories: 273

Fats: 30g

Net Carbs: 1g

Protein: 0g

Lunch

Cheddar, Bacon & Chive Cake (page 79)

Per Serving:

Calories: 573

Fats: 55g

Net Carbs: 5g

Proteins: 24g

Dinner

Buffalo Chicken Strips (refrigerate two strips, eat one third of the recipe and freeze the rest of leftovers)

Sugar Snap Peas (one portion) (page 78)

Per Serving.

Calories: 750 calories

Fats: 58.7g

Net Carbs: 9.1g

Protein: 42.3g

Day Totals.

Calories: 1596

Fats: 143.7

Net Carbs: 15.1

Protein: 66.3

Day 10

Breakfast

Bulletproof Coffee

Per Serving:

Calories: 273

Fats: 30g

Net Carbs: 1g

Protein: 0g

Lunch

Leftover Chicken Strips on Almond Bun

Per Serving:

Calories: 625

Fats: 51g

Net Carbs: 5.3g

Proteins: 49.1g

Dinner

Burger with Creamed Spinach & Almonds (eat half of the total recipe and refrigerate leftovers)

Almond Flax Bun add one tablespoon of butter to bun.

Per Serving.

Calories: 773

Fats: 59.9g

Net Carbs: 5.3g

Proteins: 49.1g

Day Totals.

Calories: 1671

Fats: 140.9

Net Carbs: 11.6

Proteins: 98.2

Day 11

Breakfast

Bulletproof Coffee

Per Serving.

Calories: 273

Fats: 30g

Net Carbs: 1g

Protein: 0g

Lunch

Leftover Burger & Spinach Salad (pages 59 and 66)

Per Serving.

Calories: 510

Fats: 42g

Net Carbs: 2.4g

Protein: 25.9g

Dinner

Bacon Mozzarella Meatballs (five meatballs freeze leftovers)

Roasted Pecan Green Beans (Eat one portion use

leftovers) (page 74)

Per Serving.

Calories: 821

Fats: 63.8g

Net Carbs: 6.7g

Protein: 54g

Day Totals.

Calories: 1604

Fats: 135.8

Net Carbs: 10.1

Protein: 79.9

Day 12

Breakfast

Bulletproof Coffee

Per Serving.

Calories: 273

Fats: 30g

Net Carbs: 1g

Protein: 0g

Lunch

Leftover Tartlets (Eat two)

Per Serving.

Calories: 481

Fats: 38.8g

Net Carbs: 4.8g

Protein: 50.3g

Dinner

Leftover Chili served with sugar snap peas (page 76)

Per Serving.

    Calories: 545

    Fats: 31.1g

    Net Carbs: 9.6g

    Protein: 53.1g

Day Totals.

    Calories: 1299

    Fats: 99.9

    Net Carbs: 15.4

    Protein: 103.4

Day 13

Breakfast

Bulletproof Coffee

Per Serving:

Calories: 273

Fats: 30g

Net Carbs: 1g

Protein: 0g

Lunch

Leftover Mozzarella Meatballs & Spinach Salad
(page 66)

Per Serving:

Calories: 641

Fats: 51.2g

Net Carbs: 3g

Protein: 35.2g

Dinner

Chicken Sausage Stir Fry Leftovers (add one quarter
cup of cheese and one tablespoon of butter) (page 64)

Per Serving.

Calories: 641

Fats: 49.3g

Net Carbs: 8.3g

Protein: 42.7g

Day Totals.

Calories: 1555

Fats: 130.5

Net Carbs: 12.3

Protein: 77.9

Day 14

Breakfast

Bulletproof Coffee

Per Serving:

Calories: 273

Fats: 30g

Net Carbs: 1g

Proteins: 0g

Lunch

Bacon, Cheddar, & Chive Mug Cake (page 79)

Per Serving:

Calories: 573

Fats: 55g

Net Carbs: 5g

Proteins: 24g

Dinner

Leftover Shrimp & Cauliflower Curry (use one tablespoon of extra butter and double serving)

(page 69)

Per Serving.

Calories: 661

Fats: 39g

Net Carbs: 11.2g

Protein: 54.8g

Day Totals.

Calories: 1507

Fats: 124

Net Carbs: 17.2

Proteins: 78.8

Chapter 3:
Recipes of Meals in Meal Planner

1) Scrambled Eggs with Cheese

Ingredients:

- one ounce of cheddar, shredded
- two tablespoons of butter
- two large eggs
- add spices of your choice
- one teaspoon of Chive, chopped

Directions:

Heat frying pan on stove add butter. Once the butter has melted add the eggs to the pan. Make sure to scramble eggs before adding to pan. Let the eggs cook on low heat. Add seasonings, chives, salt, pepper, hot sauce if you like. Add the shredded cheese and mix together.

2) Bacon Burger and Red Pepper Salad

Ingredients for Burger:

- one quarter teaspoon of onion powder
- half a teaspoon of salt
- three quarter of a teaspoon of Soy sauce
- half a teaspoon of black pepper
- half a teaspoon of garlic, minced
- one and a half teaspoons of Chives, chopped
- two tablespoons of Cheddar cheese
- two slices of bacon, chopped
- 200g of ground beef
- one quarter of a teaspoon of Worcestershire

Ingredients for Red pepper salad:

- half a teaspoon of red pepper flakes
- one and a half tablespoons of Parmesan
- two tablespoons of Ranch dressing
- three cups of spinach

Directions:

In a skillet cook your chopped bacon until it is crisp. Remove and place on paper towel. Drain the grease and save. In mixing bowl combine chopped bacon, spices, and ground beef. Mix well then form into three patties. In pan put two tablespoons of bacon fat. Once the fat is heated place patties into pan. Cook for five minutes on each side. Remove from pan let rest for five minutes. Serve with cheese, and extra bacon, and onion if this would suit your taste and then enjoy!

3) Frittata Muffins

Ingredients:

- one quarter teaspoon of salt
- half a teaspoon of pepper
- two teaspoons of Parsley, dried
- one tablespoon of butter
- half a cup of cheddar cheese
- four ounces of bacon, precooked and chopped
- half a cup of half and half cream
- eight large eggs

Directions:

Preheat the oven to 375 degrees Fahrenheit. Mix eggs with the half and half in a bowl. Add bacon and cheese, as well as spices. Add any other additional ingredients at this point. Grease the muffin tray with butter. You will yield eight muffins from this recipe. Pour the mixture into each muffin cup filling three quarters full. Put into oven for 20 minutes or until they are golden and puffy on the edges. Remove muffins from oven allow to cool for one minute. You can freeze these and heat individually.

4) Canned Chicken & Spinach Salad

Ingredients:

- three quarters of a teaspoon of curry powder, optional
- one and a half teaspoons of Dijon mustard
- one quarter of Lemon zest
- two cups of spinach
- two tablespoons of Parmesan cheese
- four tablespoons of olive oil
- one can of chicken or can use other canned meats such as turkey, or ham

Directions:

Combine all of the wet ingredients in a bowl.

Combine your meat and spinach in a bowl. Pour the wet ingredients into bowl with meat in it when you are ready to eat it.

5) Chicken Sausage Stir Fry

Ingredients:

- two teaspoons of garlic, minced
- two tablespoons of salted butter
- one quarter cup of red wine
- half a cup of tomato sauce low-carb
- half a cup of Parmesan cheese
- three cups of spinach
- three cups of broccoli florets
- four chicken sausages
- half a teaspoon of red pepper flakes

Directions:

Slice up the sausages, start to boil a pot of water on the stove. Add your sausages to a pan on high heat. Add your broccoli to the boiling water and cook for five minutes. Stir sausages until they brown on both sides. Move sausages to one side of pan then add the butter. Put garlic in the butter and saute for one minute. Mix everything together then add the broccoli. Pour tomato sauce, red wine, and red pepper flakes over. Mix together, add your spinach with salt and pepper and let cook on simmer for ten minutes. Add the Parmesan cheese to the top before serving to let it melt.

6) Spinach Salad

Ingredients:

- four cups of spinach
- four tablespoons of olive oil
- add seasonings of your choice

Directions:

Wash spinach then pat dry with paper towel to remove excess water. Chop spinach to desired size. Add olive oil with spinach in salad bowl adding seasoning of your choice toss lightly and serve.

7) Orange & Cinnamon Beef Stew

Ingredients:

- half a teaspoon of Soy sauce
- half a teaspoon of cinnamon, ground
- three quarter of a teaspoon of Thyme
- one quarter cup of orange juice
- zest of orange
- one quarter of yellow onion
- one tablespoon of coconut oil
- three quarter cup of Beef broth
- one quarter pound of ground beef
- half a teaspoon of fish sauce
- one bay leaf
- one quarter teaspoon of sage
- one quarter teaspoon of rosemary

Directions:

Cut your meat into one inch cubes and dice your veggies. Zest a whole orange. Heat coconut oil in a skillet, then add salt, pepper, and meat to skillet in batches. Do not over fill the skillet. Once you are finished browning your meat remove meat from pan and add vegetables to pan cooking for two minutes. Add orange juice to pan and other ingredients except for sage, rosemary and thyme. Let cook for a moment then transfer all ingredients to your crock pot. Let cook for three hours on high. Open your crockpot add the rest of your spices to the pot. Cook for one to two hours on high.

8) Shrimp & Cauliflower Curry

Ingredients:

- one quarter cup of butter
- one cup of coconut milk
- half a head of medium cauliflower
- one medium onion
- four cups of chicken stock
- five cups of raw spinach
- twenty-four ounces of shrimp, deveined, and peeled
- one quarter cup of heavy cream
- one fourth a teaspoon of Xanthan gum
- one fourth a teaspoon of cinnamon
- one fourth a teaspoon of cardamom
- half a teaspoon of Turmeric
- half a teaspoon of coriander
- half a teaspoon of ginger
- one teaspoon of paprika
- one teaspoon of cayenne
- one teaspoon of onion powder

- one teaspoon of chili powder
- two teaspoons of garlic powder
- one tablespoon of cumin
- one tablespoon of coconut flour
- two tablespoons of curry powder
- three tablespoons of olive oil

Directions:

Mix all the spices except for coconut flour and xanthan gum set aside. Cut up onion into slices. In pan heat olive oil and add onion slices, cook until they are soft. Add butter, heavy cream and one eighth of a teaspoon of xanthan gum and spices making sure to mix well. After about two minutes add four cups of chicken broth, and one cup of coconut milk. Stir well and cover. Cook for 30 minutes with lid on. Chop up cauliflower into small florets then add to curry. Cook for another fifteen minutes covered. Add shrimp into curry. Cook for an additional twenty minutes with the lid off. Add coconut flour and one eighth teaspoon of xanthan gum and stir well. Cook for another ten minutes with the lid off.

9) Curry Chicken Thigh

Ingredients for chicken thighs:

- one eighth of a teaspoon of cayenne pepper
- one quarter teaspoon of garlic powder
- one quarter teaspoon of paprika
- half a teaspoon of salt
- half a teaspoon of yellow curry
- one tablespoon of olive oil
- two chicken thighs
- pinch of ginger
- pinch of cinnamon
- one eighth teaspoon of coriander
- one eighth teaspoon of chili
- one eighth teaspoon of allspice

Directions:

Preheat oven to 425 degrees Fahrenheit. Mix all of the spices in a bowl. Cover a baking sheet in foil then place the chicken thighs onto it. Rub olive oil over the thighs evenly. Rub spice mixture on both sides of chicken thighs. Bake for 50 minutes. Let cool for five minutes before serving them.

Ingredients for Queso Fresco:

- half a tablespoon of olive oil
- one tablespoon of coconut oil
- one pound of Queso Fresco or Paneer cheese

Directions:

Cut cheese into cubes or thin rectangles. Heat one tablespoon of coconut oil and half a tablespoon of olive oil over high heat then add cheese. Let it cook until it is browned on one side then flip over and brown the other side. Remove from pan drain excess grease on paper towel.

10) Chorizo & Cheddar Meatballs

Ingredients:

- one tablespoon of salt
- one teaspoon of chili powder
- one teaspoon of cumin
- two large eggs
- one third of a cup of crushed pork rinds
- one cup of tomato sauce, low-carb
- one cup of cheddar cheese
- two Chorizo sausages
- one and a half pounds of ground beef

Directions:

Preheat oven to 350 degrees Fahrenheit. Break the sausage up into small pieces and mix with ground beef, ground pork rinds, cheese, spices, and eggs. Mix well then form meatballs place these on a baking tray lined with foil. Bake for 35 minutes or until the meatballs are cooked through. Spoon tomato sauce over meatball and serve.

11) Roasted Pecan Green Beans

Ingredients:

- half a teaspoon of red pepper flakes
- one teaspoon of garlic, minced
- half a lemon's zest
- two tablespoons of Parmesan cheese
- one quarter of a cup of pecans, chopped
- two tablespoons of olive oil
- half a pound of green beans

Directions:

Preheat oven to 450 then add pecans to food processor. Grind the pecans in the food processor until they are chopped nicely. Some small and large pieces. In mixing bowl mix with green beans, olive oil, Parmesan cheese, lemon zest, minced garlic, and red pepper flakes. Spread out the green beans on a foiled baking sheet. Roast beans for twenty-five minutes. Allow beans to cool for five minutes then serve!

12) Cream Cheese & Spinach Salad

Ingredients:

- one ounce of cream cheese
- three tablespoons of olive oil
- four cups of spinach

Directions:

Clean spinach then dry with paper towel to get rid of the excess water, then chop, and put into salad bowl. Add three tablespoons of olive oil and one ounce of cream cheese and lightly toss and serve.

13) Chili

Ingredients:

- two tablespoons of chili powder
- two tablespoons of olive oil
- two tablespoons of Soy sauce
- one third cup of tomato paste
- one cup of beef broth
- one green pepper
- one yellow onion
- two pounds of beef stew meat

Directions:

Half of stew meat cube up into small cubes, the other half put into food processor and make into ground beef. Chop onion and pepper up into small pieces. Combine spices together to make sauce. Saute the cubed stew beef in pan until it is browned, then transfer to slow cooker. Do the same process with the ground beef. Saute the veggies in the remaining fat for a few minutes. Add everything to slow cooker and mix well. Cook on high for two and a half hours then low for half an hour with the lid off.

14) Sugar Snap Peas

Ingredients:

- half a teaspoon of red pepper flakes
- two teaspoons of garlic, minced
- juice of half a lemon
- three cups of sugar snap peas

Directions:

Add three tablespoons of bacon fat to a pan and heat add garlic reduce heat, saute garlic for one minute. Add sugar snap peas and lemon juice and cook for two minutes. Remove and garnish with red pepper flakes and lemon zest serve and enjoy!

15) Cheddar, Bacon, & Chive Cake

Ingredients:

- one tablespoon of cheddar cheese, shredded
- two tablespoons of almond flour
- two slices of bacon
- half a teaspoon of baking powder
- two tablespoons of butter
- one egg
- two tablespoons of white cheddar, shredded
- one tablespoon of Chives, chopped
- pinch of salt
- one quarter of a teaspoon of Mrs. Dash

Directions:

Mix all ingredients in microwaveable stoneware bowl. Spray inside of bowl with non-stick cooking spray. Microwave for 70 seconds. Remove from micro and turn upside down lightly bang against plate and enjoy!

Chapter 4:
Ketogenic Recipes 16-24

The following extra recipes do not have "Per Serving charts."

16) BBQ Pulled Chicken

Makes 4 Servings

Ingredients:

- one teaspoon of fish sauce
- one teaspoon of cayenne pepper
- one teaspoon of cumin

- two teaspoons of chili powder

- one tablespoon of Soy sauce

- one tablespoon of liquid smoke

- two tablespoons of spicy brown mustard

- two tablespoons of yellow mustard

- one quarter cup of organic tomato paste

- one quarter of a cup of chicken stock

- one quarter of a cup of red wine

- one quarter cup of Stevia

- one third of a cup of salted butter

- six chicken thighs, boneless, skinless

Directions:

Mix all the ingredients except for chicken thighs. Place chicken thighs into slow cooker and pour sauce over them. Cook on low for eight hours. Take chicken and shred it down using two forks. Mix around in sauce and cook for an additional 45 minutes on high.

17) Chicken Roulade

Makes one serving

Ingredients:

- salt and pepper to taste
- 38 grams of Halloumi cheese
- one quarter of a teaspoon of garlic, minced
- zest of one quarter of a lemon
- two and one quarter of a teaspoon of olive oil
- one chicken breast
- half a tablespoon of pesto

Directions:

Pat your chicken dry getting rid of any extra moisture. Pound the chicken breast flattening. Mix one and one quarter a teaspoon of olive oil with pesto spread this mixture over chicken evenly. Add salt and pepper, garlic, and lemon zest to chicken. Add sliced Halloumi cheese to chicken breast. Roll the chicken breast up and use toothpicks to hold together.

Preheat the oven to 450 degrees Fahrenheit. Heat one tablespoon of olive oil in pan and sear each side of chicken getting it nice and brown. Bake for seven minutes until juice runs out clear.

18) Lemon Rosemary Chicken

Makes one serving

Ingredients:

- three chicken thighs, boneless, skinless
- one teaspoon of salt
- half a teaspoon of sage, dried
- three quarter of a teaspoon of rosemary, dried
- one and a half teaspoon of Thyme, fresh
- one lemon
- one and a half teaspoons of olive oil
- one and half teaspoons of garlic, minced

Directions:

Create a paste with garlic and salt grind in mortar, grinding with pestle. Add your oil and grind mixing. Dry chicken off then put into bag with mix. Coat the chicken well. Marinate the chicken overnight in fridge.

Preheat oven to 425 degrees Fahrenheit. Thinly slice lemon place slices on bottom of baking pan. Lay the chicken on top of lemon pieces. Remove the thyme leaves from stem add to chicken along with rosemary, sage, pepper and salt. Bake for 30 minutes or until the juices run clear on chicken. Remove from pan. Add the drippings to saucepan. Bring to a boil stir well. Reduce heat. Add to chicken and enjoy!

19) Bacon Wrapped Pork Tenderloin

Makes one serving with leftovers

Ingredients:

- pinch of dried sage
- pinch of cayenne
- pinch of black pepper
- one quarter of a teaspoon of rosemary, dried
- one quarter of a teaspoon of liquid smoke
- one quarter of a teaspoon of garlic, minced
- three quarter of a teaspoon of Soy sauce
- one and a half teaspoon of sugar-free Maple syrup
- one and a half teaspoons of Dijon mustard
- three slices of bacon
- half a pound of pork tenderloin

Directions:

Mix all of the wet ingredients together and dry ingredients to make a marinade. Dry pat your pork tenderloin then add to a zip-lock bag. Pour the marinade into bag, rub marinade into meat. Put into fridge for five hours.

Preheat oven to 350 degrees Fahrenheit. On a foiled baking sheet place pork and wrap in bacon. Bake for one hour, then broil for ten minutes. Cover the tenderloin with foil for ten minutes to rest. Serve and enjoy!

20) Vanilla Cookies

Makes 10 cookies

Ingredients:

- one quarter of a teaspoon of cinnamon
- half a teaspoon of salt
- half a teaspoon of baking soda
- one and a half teaspoons of vanilla
- one tablespoon + one teaspoon of instant coffee grounds
- two large eggs
- 15 drops of liquid Stevia
- half a cup of unsalted butter
- one and a half cups of almond flour
- one third a cup of Erythritol

Directions:

Preheat oven to 350 degrees Fahrenheit. Combine in a bowl, cinnamon, coffee grounds, almond flour, baking soda, and salt. In separate bowls separate whites and egg yolks. In another mixing bowl add butter and beat well add Erythritol to butter and continue to beat until it is almost white. Add your egg yolks to the butter mix until smooth. Add half of the mixed almond flour to the butter and mix. Add your vanilla extract and liquid Stevia, then add the rest of almond mix. Mix well. Beat egg whites until they are stiff, fold them into the cookie dough. Divide your cookies on a cookie sheet and make ten large cookies. Bake them for 15 minutes. Remove from oven to cooling rack allowing to cool for 15 minutes.

21) Vegetable Delight

Makes 3 Servings

Ingredients:

- half a teaspoon of red pepper flakes
- one teaspoon of pepper
- one teaspoon of salt
- six tablespoons of extra virgin olive oil
- 240g of baby Bella mushrooms
- two teaspoons of garlic, minced
- two tablespoons of pumpkin seeds
- 90g of spinach
- 90g of bell pepper, yellow
- 100g of sugar snap peas
- 115g of broccoli

Directions:

Chop all of the veggies into bite size pieces. Heat the oil then add garlic and saute for one minute, add mushrooms and allow them to soak up the oil. Then, add broccoli and mix well. Allow the broccoli to cook for a few minutes, then, add sugar snap peas. Add bell peppers, pumpkin seeds. Once cooked lay spinach on top until it is wilted, mix and serve.

22) Spicy Cakes

Makes 10 cakes

Ingredients for cake mix

- half a teaspoon of nutmeg
- half a teaspoon of cinnamon
- half a teaspoon of allspice
- one teaspoon of vanilla
- two teaspoons of baking powder
- four large eggs
- five tablespoons of water
- half a cup of salted butter
- three quarter cup of Erythritol
- two cups of almond flour
- one quarter teaspoon of clove, ground
- half a teaspoon of ginger

Ingredients for Cream Cheese Frosting:

- zest of half a lemon
- one teaspoon of vanilla extract
- three tablespoons of Erythritol

- two tablespoons of butter
- eight ounces of cream cheese

Directions:

Preheat your oven to 350 degrees Fahrenheit. In a mixing bowl add sweetener and butter. Cream them together until they are smooth. Add two eggs and continue to mix. Add last two eggs. Grind up your spices using a pestle and mortar then add to batter. Mix until smooth. Add the water and mix until it is creamy. Spray cupcake tray with non-stick cooking spray. Fill cups up with batter three quarter of the way. Place in the oven for 15 minutes. While they are baking cream together your cream cheese and your butter, sweetener, vanilla, lemon zest to make frosting. Remove the cupcakes from oven allow them to cool for 15 minutes then frost them.

23) Keto Cookies

Makes 14 cookies

Ingredients:

- one quarter of a teaspoon of baking soda
- two tablespoons of cinnamon
- one tablespoon of vanilla
- one quarter cup of sugar-free Maple syrup
- one quarter cup of coconut oil
- two cups of almond flour
- one tablespoon of Stevia

Directions:

Preheat oven to 350 degrees Fahrenheit. Mix in a bowl your baking soda, almond flour, and salt. In a separate bowl mix maple syrup, coconut oil, vanilla, and Stevia. Mix the dry ingredients into the wet ingredients mix until dough is formed. Mix cinnamon and Erythritol together until a powder is formed. Roll the dough into balls. Roll them into the cinnamon mixture, set them on baking tray that has been sprayed with non-stick cooking spray. Flatten the balls then put into oven and bake for ten minutes, remove and let cool.

24) Ginger Beef

Makes two servings

Ingredients:

- one small diced yellow onion
- two sirloin steaks
- one teaspoon of ginger, ground
- salt and pepper to taste
- four tablespoons of apple cider vinegar
- one clove of garlic, crushed
- one tablespoon of olive oil
- two small diced tomatoes

Directions:

Put oil into a large skillet, once oil is hot add steaks, brown them. Add the garlic, onion, and tomatoes once both sides of steak are browned. Cover the skillet and maintain low heat. Let simmer until all liquids have evaporated.

Chapter 5:
Recipes 25-34

25) Meatloaf

Makes 6 servings

Ingredients:

- one pound of Italian sausage
- half a teaspoon of unflavored gelatin
- two pounds of ground beef
- two tablespoons of barbecue sauce
- one quarter cup of heavy cream
- half a teaspoon of black pepper, ground
- two teaspoons of Dijon mustard

- one quarter cup of parsley leaves
- one teaspoon of salt
- one teaspoon of basil, fresh, chopped
- one tablespoon of thyme leaves
- one cup of chopped green pepper
- two large eggs
- eight ounces of white onion, chopped
- five garlic cloves, minced
- eight ounces of cream cheese, softened
- two tablespoons of butter
- half a cup of shredded parmesan cheese
- two cups of shredded cheddar cheese
- half a cup of almond flour

Directions:

Preheat the oven to 350 degrees Fahrenheit. Oil a medium sized baking dish with butter and put aside. Whisk the almond flour and parmesan cheese together in small bowl then set aside. Mix the cheddar cheese and softened cream cheese in another bowl until it has the texture of butter. In a medium skillet melt butter then add onion, garlic, and pepper. Let this cook for eight minutes until they are softened. Set aside and allow to cool.

Place remaining ingredients in a food processor for a few seconds until the vegetables are minced. In another bowl blend eggs with salt, pepper, spices, barbecue sauce, mustard, and cream. Add the gelatin on top and leave if for five minutes. Mix onion mixture and set aside. Mix the sausage and beef. Put the meatloaf mixture back into the large mixing bowl adding egg mixture, mix well. Add the almond flour mixture mixing until the meat no longer sticks. Cover a cookie sheet with wax paper placing meat mixture on there to form a slab shape. Spread the slab with cream cheese mixture. Roll the meat up covering the ends to protect the cheese mixture from spilling out. Let bake until browned for 30 minutes. Slice and serve.

26) Pork Chops

Makes four servings

Ingredients:

- half a teaspoon of mixed spice
- half a tablespoon of chili paste
- one and a half teaspoons of soy sauce
- one tablespoon of almond flour
- one tablespoon of sugar-free ketchup
- four garlic cloves
- one tablespoon of fish sauce
- one medium star anise
- one stalk of lemon grass, peeled, and diced
- four pork chops
- one teaspoon of sesame oil
- half a teaspoon of peppercorns

Directions:

Roll on pork chops with rolling pin that is wrapped in wax paper. Cut garlic cloves into halves then set aside. Grind the peppercorns and anise until they form a fine powder using a mortar and pestle. Add the garlic and lemongrass making smooth mixture. Add soy sauce and fish sauce, mixed spice, sesame oil, and mix well. Place pork chops on a tray then coat with the marinade at room temperature. Cover for two hours.

Preheat pan and lightly coat the pork chops with almond flour. Place them into pan and turn once when they have seared on both sides. Cut chops up into small strips. Make sauce by stirring in ketchup and chili paste. Serve with mashed potatoes or crisp garlic parmesan green beans.

27) Baked Salmon

Makes Two Servings

Ingredients:

- two salmon fillets
- one tablespoon of lemon juice
- one tablespoon of parsley, freshly chopped
- one teaspoon of salt
- one teaspoon of pepper, ground
- six tablespoons of olive oil
- one teaspoon of dried basil
- two cloves of garlic, minced
- one teaspoon of dill, dried

Directions:

In a glass bowl mix up the marinade using light olive oil, lemon juice, parsley, dill, salt, garlic, and pepper. In a medium sized baking dish put the salmon fillets in with skin side down. Spread the marinade on fillets. Put into the fridge for an hour.

Preheat oven to 375 degrees Fahrenheit. Place fillets inside foil and seal placing in glass baking dish. Bake until the fillets are nice and flaky in texture.

28) Fried Chicken

Makes 4 Servings

Ingredients:

- half a cup of parmesan cheese, shredded
- one eighth teaspoon of coarse black pepper
- half a teaspoon of onion powder
- one cup of crushed pork rinds
- one tablespoon of oat fiber
- three quarter of a cup of plain whey protein
- a quarter cup of heavy cream
- two large eggs
- four chicken breasts, skinned, boneless
- half inch deep of hot coconut oil
- one quarter cup of water

Directions:

Shake all of the dry ingredients in a plastic bag. Mix the cream, water, and eggs in a large bowl, add chicken. Make sure to coat chicken well by turning several times or so. Remove each piece and coat with the seasoned flour. Heat the oil on high arrange pieces of chicken in pan then coat the other pieces and repeat process. Cook until the chicken is brown on both sides. Remove and allow to drain on a piece of paper towel.

29) Avocados & Shrimps

Makes one serving

Ingredients:

- one teaspoon of unsweetened coconut, shredded
- one tablespoon of coconut milk
- half a teaspoon of hot sauce
- half a tablespoon of organic peanut butter
- half an avocado
- one cup of shrimps, deveined, peeled

Directions:

Spray the saucepan with olive oil spray put on to medium temperature. Pour the coconut milk, peanut butter, hot sauce mix. Add shrimps and saute for about five minutes, until the shrimp turn pink. Slice the avocado into small pieces, put shrimp mixture on serving plates and top with avocado and shredded coconut.

30) Keto Style Casserole

Makes two servings

Ingredients:

- one- eight ounce package of cream cheese
- one can of sauerkraut, drained
- two cups of Swiss cheese, shredded
- half a pound of corned beef, diced
- two tablespoons of pickle brine
- half a teaspoon of caraway seeds
- half a cup of low-sugar ketchup
- half a cup of mayonnaise

Directions:

Preheat oven to 350 degrees Fahrenheit. Melt the mayonnaise, ketchup, and cream cheese, over low heat in a saucepan. Slice the corned beef diced bits. Add one and a half cups of Swiss cheese, corned beef, and drained sauerkraut once mixture is melted. Mix until it is well blended. Remove from heat and add pickle juice, and pinch of garlic salt to taste. Put into oiled dish add remaining Swiss cheese on top. Sprinkle caraway seeds on top to garnish. Put into oven for 20 minutes or until cheese is melted.

31) Chipotle & Asparagus Mayonnaise

Makes four Servings

Ingredients:

- half a cup of mayonnaise
- one Chipotle chili
- one teaspoon of adobe sauce
- two pounds of asparagus

Directions:

Remove the ends of asparagus then put them into a microwaveable casserole dish. Add a few tablespoons of water, then cover with plastic wrap. Let heat in microwave for five minutes. Put your Chipotle chili and mayonnaise into food processor, add a teaspoon of adobo sauce. Blend until smooth. Serve.

32) Creamed Spinach

Makes two servings

Ingredients:

- three tablespoons of butter
- two tablespoons of cream cheese
- ten ounces of spinach, frozen, chopped
- salt and pepper to taste

Directions:

Place spinach in a microwaveable bowl add four tablespoons of water then cover. Cook in micro for eight minutes. Stir and then put back in for another four minutes. After done pour into a strainer in sink. Press with spoon to remove excess water. Transfer the spinach to a bowl and add the cream cheese, and butter. Stir until it becomes smooth. Add salt and pepper to taste and divide onto two serving plates enjoy!

33) Low-carb Hawaiian Pizza

Makes two individual size Pizzas

Ingredients:

- two medium sized low-carb pita breads
- two ounces of mozzarella cheese per pita
- three tablespoons of tomato sauce
- one dash of garlic powder
- dash of ground pepper
- two slices of bacon
- one tablespoon of roasted red peppers
- one handful of spinach
- half a cup of artichokes
- half a cup of black olives, pitted, sliced
- half a cup of unsweetened pineapple, diced
- one cup of ham

Directions:

Preheat the oven to 450 degrees Fahrenheit. Spray the pitas with cooking spray put into preheated oven for about two minutes. Mix tomato sauce with garlic, black pepper, add to bread when removed from oven. Add cheese. Spread with olive oil and other ingredients and let bake for another five minutes.

34) Egg Whites & Beef Scramble

Makes two servings

Ingredients:

- salt and pepper to taste
- two Italian tomatoes
- four small tomatoes
- half a cup of red peppers
- eight egg whites
- two cups of baby spinach
- one pound of extra lean ground beef
- one tablespoon of basil, fresh, chopped

Directions:

Heat a pan sprayed with olive oil over medium heat then add beef to hot pan. Break beef into smaller pieces while cooking. Once it is cooked put into bowl and set aside. Beat the egg whites and pour them over the cooked meat. Saute the spinach, tomatoes, peppers, and basil, place on top of meat once finished sauteing. Serve hot.

Chapter 6:
Recipes 35-45

35) Cauliflower, Cheese, & Bacon Quiche

Makes four servings

Ingredients:

- half a cup of heavy cream
- salt and pepper to taste
- two cups of cheddar, or Colby jack cheese, shredded
- six eggs
- one tablespoon of butter

- four ounces of bacon, cooked, crumbled
- four ounces of white onion, minced
- two ounces of green pepper, minced
- two pounds of raw cauliflower

Directions:

Cut the cauliflower into small pieces, including the core. Bring a large pan of water to boil and lightly salt. On medium heat add the cauliflower and cook until it is tender. This should take about 30 minutes. Drain the cauliflower with colander then set aside. Melt the butter and saute the bell pepper and onions over medium heat. Mince cauliflower when it has cooled. Press out the excess water from the cauliflower, using paper towel. Press the cauliflower into a sprayed baking pan that is coated with non-stick cooking spray. Dip bacon into the onion, pepper mixture. Spoon it over the cauliflower. Add the shredded cheese to the top. Beat eggs, and blend them with the cream and spices until they are turned frothy. Pour over the cauliflower. Put in oven for 35 minutes or until the top is golden.

36) Garlic & Cheddar Biscuits

Makes 37 biscuits

Ingredients:

- five tablespoons of butter
- two and a half cups of almond flour, divided
- six ounces of Colby jack cheese, shredded
- three quarter of a teaspoon of xanthum gum
- one teaspoon of sea salt
- two teaspoons of garlic powder
- one teaspoon of baking soda
- eight ounces of cream cheese
- two large eggs

Directions:

Preheat oven to 325 degrees Fahrenheit. Spread parchment paper on cookie sheet. Place one cup of shredded cheese and almond flour in a food processor. Finely ground then set aside. Put the butter and cream cheese into a stoneware bowl put into oven for a few minutes until the butter starts to melt. Remove and whisk until it is smooth. Beat in the eggs until the mixture turns smooth. Blend in garlic, and xanthium gum, baking soda, and salt. Mix almond flour and cheese mixture and egg mixture. Add the remaining almond flour and stir until well mixed and forms a dough. Use a tablespoon to scoop the dough then place on the cookie sheet, making one inch gaps between them. Bake for 25 minutes or until golden brown, remove and allow to cool for ten minutes.

37) Chicken Noodle Soup

Makes two servings

Ingredients:

- one teaspoon of chicken bouillon concentrate
- one package of tofu shirataki noodles
- four tablespoons of shredded carrot
- two cups of chicken broth
- two tablespoons of chopped onion
- five tablespoons of diced celery
- four tablespoons of coconut oil

Directions:

Melt the coconut oil in a pan over low heat. Add veggies and saute for about five minutes. Add the chicken bouillon and broth then mix and bring to a simmer. Reduce the heat and cover allowing it to simmer for an additional 20 minutes. Drain your shirataki noodles, put them into a microwaveable bowl. Cook on high for two minutes and drain them again. Separate the noodles. Add noodles to soup and let simmer for another few minutes before serving.

38) Pecans & Strawberries

Makes one serving

Ingredients:

- one large strawberry
- one tablespoon of pecans
- one tablespoon of french vanilla liquid Stevia
- one third of a cup of sour cream

Directions:

In a small skillet stir the pecans over medium low heat for a few minutes to make them crispier. Remove the pecans from the heat. Sweeten sour cream with Stevia in a small serving bowl, mix well. Slice strawberry put on top along with pecans and enjoy!

39) Chocolate, Macadamia, Peanut Butter Treats

Makes six treats

Ingredients:

- three teaspoons of Stevia
- half a cup of Macadamia nuts
- four tablespoons of natural creamy peanut butter
- one tablespoon of heavy whipping cream
- nine tablespoons of organic butter
- five ounces of dark chocolate

Directions:

Microwave the butter and chocolate for a few seconds until melted. Add the rest of the ingredients except the Macadamia nuts. Blend until smooth. Stir in the Macadamia nuts, then pour two teaspoons into each baking cup. Store in the freezer. Eat frozen or allow to warm for a few minutes.

40) Jalapeno Peppers & Bacon

Makes one serving

Ingredients:

- one and a half ounces of cream cheese
- two slices of bacon
- two jalapeno peppers, fresh
- half a teaspoon of garlic, minced

Directions:

Remove the stems and seeds from the peppers. Mix garlic well into the cream cheese in small bowel then divide the cream cheese into two, stuffing the peppers with it. Roll the peppers in the bacon and seal with toothpicks. Then you can either broil or grill until the bacon is cooked.

41) Stuffed Mushrooms

Makes a good Appetizer or Snack

Ingredients:

- Paprika to garnish
- eight ounces of Boursin cheese
- half a cup of low-sodium chicken broth
- one pound of mushrooms
- one teaspoon of garlic, minced
- half a teaspoon of Parsley

Directions:

Preheat oven to 350 degrees Fahrenheit. Remove the stems from mushrooms save to use with other dish. Fill Mushrooms with Boursin and place onto baking pan. Fill bottom of the pan with chicken broth. Sprinkle top with paprika, parsley and top with small amount of minced garlic.

42) Deviled Eggs

Makes two servings

Ingredients:

- one teaspoon of cumin
- one teaspoon of paprika
- few drops of hot sauce
- one tablespoon of mayonnaise
- one teaspoon of honey mustard
- salt and pepper to taste
- parsley as garnish
- half a teaspoon of cayenne pepper

Directions:

Remove the yolk from hard boiled eggs. Mash the yolk in a bowl with other ingredients, until well blended. Fill eggs with mixture sprinkle top with paprika. Refrigerate until ready to serve.

43) Bacon, Eggs, & Veggies

Makes four servings

Ingredients:

- half a cup of Colby jack cheese, shredded
- four large organic eggs
- half of a white onion, chopped
- half a cup of cauliflower or broccoli, chopped
- half a cup of celery, finely chopped
- eight slices of pemale bacon, sliced
- one carrot, peeled into fine strips.
- one tablespoon of butter

Directions:

Slice the bacon into small thin strips. Put butter in skillet over medium heat, once it has melted add the bacon and veggies. Saute the bacon and veggies in the butter for about 20 minutes while stirring occasionally. Spread the mixture evenly over the bottom of skillet. Divide into quarter sections, break an egg over each separate section. Cook until eggs are set. You can cover the pan to cook the eggs thoroughly. Add cheese just before eggs have completely set.

44) Avocado, Bacon, Turkey Salad

Makes one serving

Ingredients for dressing:

- one teaspoon of Dijon mustard
- salt and pepper to taste
- half a teaspoon of garlic, minced
- one tablespoon of apple cider vinegar
- one teaspoon of fresh lemon juice
- one tablespoon of extra virgin olive oil

Ingredients for salad:

- two cups of romaine lettuce, coarsely chopped
- half an avocado, diced
- 30 grams of blue cheese
- two hard boiled eggs
- 100 grams of ham
- four grape tomatoes
- extra virgin olive oil cooking spray
- two slices of turkey bacon

Directions:

Cut ham into small cubes then heat in pan coated with olive oil spray for a few minutes. Slice up the hard boiled eggs. Place the lettuce in empty serving bowl. Add avocado, grape tomatoes, turkey bacon, blue cheese, eggs and ham. Spread dressing evenly over the top and enjoy!

45) Guacamole

Makes a good Snack or Appetizer

Ingredients:

- half a tablespoon of cilantro, minced
- dash of hot sauce
- one quarter of lime, fresh
- one tablespoon of olive oil
- one teaspoon of garlic, minced
- one avocado, ripe
- one tablespoon of red onion, minced

Directions:

Mush up avocado, add onion, and garlic, mix well.
Add rest of ingredients and mix well then serve.

Conclusion

The ketogenic diet is becoming a more popular and is certainly one of the best healthy ways to quickly lose weight. It was originally designed for people that have been battling with epilepsy. But it is also beneficial for anyone that is looking to lose weight, or get their diabetes under control, or for those looking for a healthier diet. I hope that you will find the meal planner and recipes helpful to you in your personal journey towards better health. You have made the right first step towards this goal just by downloading this book. I wish you great health and well-being, by starting on the ketogenic diet you will be well on your way to achieving these!

Thanks again for downloading my book if you have a moment in between cooking up a great ketogenic recipe I would greatly appreciate if you could take a moment to leave a review for my book thanks and good luck with your new healthy eating habits!

Finally, if you enjoyed this book, then I'd like to ask you for a big favor, would you be kind enough to leave a review for this book on Amazon? It'd be greatly appreciated!

Book 2
My Spiralized Cookbook: 40 Delicious Spiralized Recipes for Optimum Health, Weight loss & Wellness You Need To Know

Introduction

Do you want to learn 40 healthy and delicious spiralized recipes for weight loss and optimum health?

If you are looking for healthy new recipes that not only offer you good foods with health benefits but also look appealing to the eye with the way they are presented you should really enjoy delving into this cookbook.

For those who are looking to try something different in how they prepare and serve their meals you will enjoy trying the great recipes offered in this cookbook. It can get boring sometimes having the same old same old kind of meals. Perhaps you are trying to find a way to keep your family interested in eating healthier food choices. If you can present them with a new meal based on a spiral slicer recipe then I am sure they will be delighted with the presentation and the taste of the meal. It can be trying at times to get your loved ones to eat healthier foods but just keep in mind that you must show your children by example. You are the one that is in control of what foods come into your household.

Sit down and talk with your family and explain to them that you want to present healthier meals to them because you love and care about them and want them to be healthy and strong. You will be surprised how understanding your children can be when you explain the health concerns you have when choosing certain kinds of foods. They will be more willing to except new foods if you explain to them the benefits that these new healthy foods will provide for them. Educating your children on making healthy food choices and what they consist of will make it easier for you to get them on board with a healthier diet plan. I hope you and your family enjoy the spiral slicer recipes gathered in this cookbook!

Chapter 1:
Finding the Right Spiral Slicer Tool for You

I must confess I am someone that loves my kitchen gadgets, so I was immediately drawn when I started to see spiral vegetable slicers, spiral cutters, or whatever else you want to call them—I was hooked, I knew I wanted one of those. I am trying to offer my family healthier food choices so when I thought that I could get more vegetables into my family's diet I was attracted to this notion. If I could present more healthy foods to my family in a new way then why not?

To be honest for me the thought of adding more cups full of broccoli to my daily diet did not appeal to me, but if I could add more veggies into my families diet by replacing pasta with vegetables and making them into more tasty side dishes or entrees was something I was going to check out and give it a try.

All of the Julienne and spiral slicer peelers all appeared to have fun varieties of spiral slices that you could make. The Mandoline even offered an array of cuts that I could use in making my vegetable dishes with. I now had a goal or mission if you will to find a spiral cutter that would suit my needs best. I was on the search for this gadget that would help me to reduce the carbohydrates in my family's diet.

I found the one that would work for me—more about my choice of spiral slicer later. I began to do some experimenting. Most of the recipes I tried at first were designed to substitute pastas in a dish with zucchini noodles. They were really easy and quick to make and they tasted great—my family loved them!

I wanted to find other ways to use my newly acquired kitchen gadget. So I decided I was going to liven up a salad. I began thinking what if I could use favorite classic dishes but just give them a bit of an upgrade in the presentation department by using spiral veggies in them.

I began to realize that there was a lot more I could do with my new gadget than I had originally realized. I started to try different combinations of fruits and veggies some were more favored than others. But in the process I ended up coming up with side dishes, main dishes that I wanted to share with others. I served my dishes to friends and family asking their honest opinions of the dishes so I ended up with the best of the best now gathered here in these pages. I was sure my husband might grumble a bit when I made some changes to some of his favorite meals but to my surprise he enjoyed the new versions. He was also happy because they were healthier as he wants to eat better to help control his diabetes.

So here in this cookbook is my own collection of my favorite spiral veggie dishes and those of my loved ones too! In this cookbook my goal was to bring together new recipes for main dishes, salads, soups, and side dishes that are a more healthier and appealing choice in order to help us to eat more vegetables. Included are dishes for vegetarians, low carbohydrate diets, gluten-free diets, also a good variety of fish, meat, and poultry dishes too.

There is recipes that will make great side dishes and salads that will go with any type of meal that you are serving. Learning to expand the traditional boundaries of vegetables is going to make your options on preparing your meals so much more allowing you to serve in so many different ways!

You are going to find that a spiral slicer is going to add so much more to your experience of eating fruits and vegetables, this cookbook will help to guide you through ways that you can present your family with meals that are healthy and can be prepared quickly. But most of all you will please your friends and family with the great tastes of your meals. Enjoy exploring the world of spiralizing your foods!

If you are trying to find a more tantalizing way to serve your fruits and vegetables then you are ready to give spiralizing a try. You are going to be creating meals that are healthy, quick to prepare but most of all are great tasting! You can use a spiral cutter to cut your veggies and fruits for soups, salads, main dishes, and sides much quicker.

Cutting long slices are appealing for a healthy alternative to pasta. The shapes are also ideal for soups, salads, stir fries, and side dishes. You can also use your spiral cutter to make garnishes for your appetizers and many other dishes.

Spiral slicers, Julienne Peelers, Mandolines, Spiral Slicers, and other Veggie Cutters. Each of these are used to cut veggies and fruit into thin, long, slices that are extremely stream lined.

There is a vast number of *Spiral Slicers* in the market today to choose from. You can find them in kitchen stores, or big retail stores, Amazon, etc.

There is basically three different types of spiral slicers and amongst these are many brand names.

Spiral slicer is the first type it is the biggest or largest. It features three to four different sizes of cutting blades. You are able to cut from spaghetti size noodles, to fettuccine, to wider egg noodle sized pasta.

Advantages: It has a large base with suction cups that hold to your cupboard; it has a hand crank that keeps your fingers away from the blades it also gives you more leverage for turning denser veggies.

Disadvantages: This is a large gadget due to its overall

size if you have limited kitchen space this would not be a good choice. Some of the models have platforms extending beyond the blades while others do not. It is nice to have this so that your veggies you are cutting can drop right into bowl meaning less cleanup for you. You need to take caution when changing the blades or cleaning them.

Midsize Spiral slicer is the second type. It usually has four different size cutting blades. It is more compact than the previous type.

Small Spiral slicer is the third type it is a handheld kitchen tool. It has two blades one for thick pasta another for thin pasta. This is a good choice if you only want to use it to make spaghetti sized noodles. It is a good compact tool for this purpose.

Julienne Peelers these are kitchen tools that have been around for a very long time. You can find these at most stores that sell small kitchen gadgets. They come with various blades on different brands and types. Make sure you choose one that has ultra-sharp serrated blades that will be ideal for the types of size cuts that you want to make. These are small enough that you can keep them in a utensil drawer.

Mandolines are another kitchen tool that have been around for a long time. They too can be found at most stores that sell small kitchen gadgets. These are really good to use if you are cutting eggplant into wide lasagna noodle size slices. Look for a Mandoline that offers multiple size blades and a thickness adjuster. Make sure that it has a food holder and protects your fingers from being cut. You can also find Mandolines that have clamps on them so you can secure them to the side of a bowl.

Other Spiral Vegetable Cutters. If you have a food processor or a stand mixer with the ability to add attachments you can also use these appliances to cut your veggies and fruits. There is attachments that can do shredding, grinding, and julienne cuts. Depending on the spiral slicer that you choose will have an effect on what your choices are for spiral sizes.

Garlic Press: A garlic press is not a necessity but you will find they are handy to have when you need to mince some garlic they do the job well. They are also much easier to use than a knife for this job.

Strainer: It is good to have a strainer in your kitchen especially when you are using a lot of foods that need to be washed before use, and also strained of excess water. You can also use some paper towel to help you to get rid of any excess water if you want to speed the process along.

Vegetable Peeler: It will really help you when you need to peel your veggies and fruit it just makes this process so much easier when preparing the foods.

Large Sharp Knife: You need a good large sharp knife to help you to cut up denser larger veggies and it well help to cut the ends off your produce.

Chapter 2:
Stocking Up On Spiralizing Supplies

The great thing about adding more veggies to your diet is you are going to be trading in the traditional pasta for your spiralizing veggies that is going to eliminate gluten, lower your calories, and reduce your intake of carbohydrates.

Vegetables & Fruits

Make sure to use good quality and freshest produce that you can find. You want to make sure that your meals are going to be the best they can be so strive for quality foods to be included in your meals. Fully ripened fruits and vegetables should always be used when preparing your meals. You do not want to use produce that is either over-ripe or under-ripe. By choosing produce that is in season in your area you will get best results from this choice. Not only will they taste better if grown locally but they often are sold at very good prices especially at the local farmer's markets. Zucchini is a very popular choice of veggie amongst those that like to spiralize their meals. It is the most popular choice to substitute pasta in recipes. But there is also many other choices you can try to make delicious healthy meals for your family. I find some of the best veggies to spiralize are: zucchini, sweet potatoes, summer squash, cucumbers, carrots, russet potatoes, eggplant, cabbage, beets turnips, parsnips, onions, radishes. Fruits that are ideal are apples and pears.

Condiments & Broths

Using beef, chicken, or vegetable broths are wonderful for simmering veggie noodles in. Broths will add a nice deep flavor to your meats and soups. You can buy containers of broth, bouillon cubes, or make it from scratch.

Having a variety of condiments will help to add some zing to your flavoring of your meals try using: honey, Worcestershire sauce, and Dijon Mustard, honey mustard. These items will certainly come in handy when you are preparing your meals they will help to give the flavor of your meals a nice boost.

Oils & Vinegars

Using oil is one of the standard ingredients for many of these recipes you can choose from the best oils that I would suggest are extra virgin olive oil and coconut oil. Vinegar is a great staple to have on hand you will be able to use this in many of your meals. There is an assortment of different vinegars to choose from my personal favorite is apple cider vinegar.

Herbs & Seasoning

When you are adding dried herbs and seasoning to your meals remember that a small amount will go a long way in flavoring your foods. Make sure to follow the guidelines in the recipes for the amounts to use so that you get the proper consistency and flavor. You may want to adjust the amounts to your personal taste once you become familiar with making the recipes you can tweak them to suit your tastes.

Ingredients List

Make sure that when you are planning to make a certain recipe that you write a list of the ingredients that are needed before you go shopping, then make sure to bring your list. I myself am great at writing lists but when I get to the grocery store I often realize I have forgotten my list. Before leaving the house give yourself a check over to make sure you have your shopping supplies such as list and shopping bags. When you are using fresh fruits and veggies in a recipe you should buy them when you want to make the dish or no more than two to three days previous to preparing dish for the best results. Make sure to have your veggies prepped and ready before you begin to cook so that you are not left with foods that are overcooked and soggy. Add your ingredients in the order that they are listed within the recipe directions.

Tips for Best Results

You should make sure to read the manual that you will receive with your spiral slicer so that you assemble it properly and know the most effective way to use it. Try and choose thick, firm, and straight veggies and fruits. Do not choose veggies that are too big as they will be hard for you to handle and they may not fit into your spiral slicer. Try and use veggies that have little to no seeds in them. If they are a veggie that does have seeds pick the thinner ones as they will have less seeds. Make sure you are using good quality produce and wash and dry them properly before using. When putting into your spiral slicer make sure they are as straight as you can place them. When you are cooking veggies it is better if you do not overcrowd the pot or pan you are cooking in. Clean your tools right after using to keep them in the best condition.

Safety Tips

The blades are very sharp on these slicers so take extra care when washing and handling them. Make sure that you dry your blades after washing to prevent them from tarnishing or rusting. Now it is time to begin using your spiral slicer and getting creative in the kitchen in a healthy way!

Chapter 3:
Spiralized Salads

To begin your adventure into the world of spiral slicer meals here is a wide variety of soups and salad recipes I am sure you are going to enjoy preparing these healthy fun dishes!

1. Thai Salad & Peanut Lime Ginger Dressing

Servings: 4

Ingredients:

- three tablespoons of fresh cilantro
- one lime wedge
- two and a half tablespoons of unsalted peanuts
- one English cucumber, sliced
- one quarter cup of finely shredded fresh ginger
- two yellow beets, spiralized
- two large carrots, spiralized
- one cup of Napa cabbage chopped
- four tablespoons of Peanut Lime Ginger Dressing

Peanut Ginger Dressing Ingredients:

- half a cup of extra virgin olive oil
- one tablespoon of Stevia
- two tablespoons of coconut milk
- one quarter cup of shredded fresh ginger

- one tablespoon of apple cider vinegar
- two tablespoons of lime juice
- two tablespoons of peanut butter smooth
- two tablespoons of cilantro
- one teaspoon of minced garlic

Directions for Dressing:

In a blender puree all of the ingredients except for the olive oil. When blender is running add the oil in an easy stream until the dressing is nice and smooth.

Directions:

Put the cabbage in a large serving bowl. Using either a julienne or a spiral slicer, spiralize the yellow beets, and carrots into spaghetti size noodles. Add these to the top of the cabbage. Drizzle on top with Peanut Ginger Dressing. Add peanuts, cilantro, cucumbers, and lime as garnish and enjoy!

2. Kohlrabi Salad

Servings: 4

Ingredients:

- two tablespoons of balsamic dressing
- one tablespoon of dried cranberries
- one green apple, spiralized
- two tablespoons of walnuts chopped
- one kohlrabi peeled and spiralized
- two cups of baby arugula
- one cup of diced feta cheese
- garnish with sesame seeds

Directions:

Place the arugula in a large bowl, using either a julienne peeler or a spiral slicer to spiralize the kohlrabi and the green apple into spaghetti size strands. Add these to the top of the arugula. Then add diced feta cheese, dried cranberries, walnuts and dressing. Then garnish with sesame seeds and serve.

3. Tomatoes & Mango with Curry Zucchini Pasta

Servings: 2

Ingredients:

- half a mango cut into cubes
- six cherry tomatoes cut in half
- one zucchini, spiralized
- two tablespoons of extra virgin olive oil
- two cups of baby spinach
- one tablespoon of fresh basil chopped
- two tablespoons of curry powder
- sea salt
- fresh parsley for garnish
- slivered almonds for garnish

Directions:

Using a spiral slicer or julienne peeler, spiralize the zucchini into spaghetti size noodles in a bowl. Add the sea salt, olive oil, basil, and curry powder to zucchini. Toss gently and then set aside.

On a plate add baby spinach, tomatoes, and mango, top with zucchini mixture then add parsley and almonds as garnish.

4. Asian Sweet Potato Salad

Servings: 4

Ingredients:

- eight green onions finely sliced
- two tablespoons of sesame seeds
- two cups of kale remove the stems
- one red bell pepper thinly sliced
- five ounces of portabella mushrooms thinly sliced
- two tablespoons of sugar-free maple syrup
- one yellow onion thinly sliced
- one quarter cup of tamari sauce or low-sodium soy sauce
- three and a half tablespoons of extra virgin olive oil divided
- three large carrots, spiralized
- two large sweet potatoes peeled and spiralized
- one teaspoon of minced garlic

Directions:

Using a julienne peeler or a spiral slicer, spiralize the sweet potatoes into spaghetti size noodles. Spiralize you carrots cut into four to four and a half inch lengths and set aside. In a deep skillet toss around sweet potato noodles with two teaspoons of oil cooking over medium-low heat until slightly softened. Remove noodles from heat. In a small bowl combine the soy sauce, maple syrup, garlic and two tablespoons of oil. Blend this well. Add to the pan with the sweet potatoes and gently toss. Remove to serving plate and add sesame seeds and green onions.

5. Bitter Sweet Cucumber Salad

Servings: 4

Ingredients:

- half of a red onion sliced and quartered
- three English cucumbers, spiralized
- three quarter cup of apple cider vinegar
- one and a half tablespoons of Stevia
- one tablespoon of sesame seeds
- fresh parsley finely chopped for garnish

Directions:

Spiralize your cucumbers into wide noodles using either a julienne peeler or a spiral slicer. Collect the noodles into a bowl. Add vinegar, red onion, Stevia and one quarter cup of water. Cover the bowl tightly and refrigerate the noodles for at least two hours stir occasionally. One the salad is well chilled then top with sesame seeds and parsley.

6. Curried White Kidney Beans & Zucchini Salad

Servings: 4

Ingredients:

- two zucchini, spiralized
- two large carrots, spiralized
- one green cabbage cut into thin strips
- one can of white kidney beans drained and rinsed
- one quarter cup of fresh cilantro chopped
- four green onions sliced
- one red bell pepper thinly sliced
- pinch of red chili flakes
- pinch of fresh ground pepper
- pinch of sea salt
- one third cup of tahini
- three tablespoons of lime juice
- four tablespoons of sugar-free maple syrup
- one tablespoon of ground ginger
- one tablespoon of curry powder

Directions:

In a large bowl add ground ginger, maple syrup, curry powder, lime juice, and tahini. Mix these ingredients well add a bit of water if needed. Using a spiral slicer or julienne peeler spiralize your zucchini, and carrots into spaghetti size noodles. In a large bowl, add cabbage, bell pepper, noodles, green onions, cilantro, and white kidney beans. Add your dressing and toss to coat. You can season with red chili flakes and salt and pepper.

7. Apple, Beet, & Radish Slaw

Servings: 4

Ingredients:

- one red beet, spiralized
- one bunch of radishes, spiralized
- one green medium sized apple, spiralized
- one quarter cup of apple cider vinegar
- Romaine lettuce leaves
- pinch of sea salt
- two teaspoons of finely grated orange zest
- two tablespoons of fresh ginger finely grated
- one teaspoon of basil
- one quarter cup of cilantro
- two tablespoons of low-sodium soy sauce

Directions:

Spiralize your apple, beet, and radishes into spaghetti sized noodles using a julienne peeler or a spiral slicer. Add these ingredients to a large bowl along with vinegar, soy sauce, cilantro, basil, ginger, and orange zest. Toss your salad add a pinch of sea salt if you desire then allow it to rest for five minutes before serving. Place Romaine leaves on top of plates then put the slaw on top of them and serve.

8. Sweet Potato Walnut Salad

Servings: 4

Ingredients:

- three sweet potatoes peeled and spiralized
- half a cup of extra virgin olive oil divided
- sea salt
- half a cup of scallions chopped
- two tablespoons of apple cider vinegar
- one teaspoon of Dijon Mustard
- one teaspoon of minced garlic
- half a cup of feta cheese crumbled
- one bunch of baby spinach leaves
- half a cup of walnuts chopped

Directions:

Preheat your oven to 425 degrees Fahrenheit. Using a spiral slicer or julienne peeler spiralize your sweet potatoes into spaghetti size noodles. Toss in two tablespoons of oil with your sweet potatoes and sea salt. Place on a large roasting pan and cover with foil. Roast for about 15 minutes or until golden brown and turn occasionally. During the last five minutes put your walnuts on a small baking sheet and add them to the oven. Put your spinach into a large bowl with feta cheese, and scallions. Put the remaining olive oil, mustard, vinegar, garlic into jar and shake well to mix and blend ingredients. Pour this over your spinach mixture then add the potatoes and walnuts on top and serve.

9. Spicy Cucumber Salad

Servings: 6

Ingredients:

- four cucumbers, spiralized
- two carrots, spiralized
- one teaspoon of garlic minced
- one teaspoon of fresh ginger grated
- one teaspoon of raw honey
- half a tablespoon of apple cider vinegar
- one tablespoon of extra virgin olive oil
- one quarter cup of low-sodium soy sauce
- sesame seeds to garnish
- cilantro for garnish
- cayenne pepper sauce for spice level you want

Directions:

Spiralize your carrots and zucchini into spaghetti size noodles then place the noodles into a bowl. In a mixing bowl whisk together the lime juice, honey, ginger, oil, vinegar, and cayenne pepper sauce. Add the dressing to the noodles and toss gently adding cilantro to garnish and sesame seeds.

10. Zucchini & Dandelion Salad

Servings: 6

Ingredients:

- two zucchini, spiralized
- four cups of Dandelion leaves
- one cup of cherry tomatoes halved
- one teaspoon of extra virgin olive oil
- two tablespoons of balsamic vinaigrette
- sea salt
- fresh ground pepper
- half a cup of feta cheese crumbled
- four tablespoons of slivered almonds for garnish

Directions:

Spiralize your zucchini into spaghetti size noodles using a spiral slicer or julienne peeler. Add the Dandelion leaves, feta cheese, olive oil, balsamic vinaigrette. Sprinkle on top with slivered almonds and serve.

11. Tomatoes, Carrots & Zucchini Salad

Servings: 4

Ingredients:

- one quarter cup of apple cider vinegar
- quarter cup of grape tomatoes halved
- one quarter cup of coconut oil melted
- one teaspoon of minced garlic
- one teaspoon of Stevia
- half a teaspoon of sea salt
- two zucchini, spiralized
- one large carrot, spiralized
- two tablespoons of fresh basil chopped
- half a cup of Parmesan cheese shaved

Directions:

Spiralize your carrot and zucchini into spaghetti size noodles using a spiral slicer or julienne peeler. In a bowl combine carrot, zucchini, and tomatoes. In a container with lid combine oil, vinegar, garlic, Stevia, garlic seal with lid and shake well. Pour the dressing over the noodles and toss lightly then allow it to sit for ten minutes, add Parmesan and basil then, serve.

12. Spicy Mango & Cucumber Salad

Servings: 4

Ingredients:

- three cucumbers, spiralized
- two tablespoons of extra virgin olive oil
- sea salt
- two cups of kale greens
- half a mango cubed
- two tablespoons of curry powder
- fresh chopped cilantro
- two tablespoons of slivered almonds

Directions:

Spiralize your cucumbers into spaghetti size noodles into a bowl using a spiral slicer or a julienne peeler. Add oil, cilantro, and sea salt to cucumber. Add the amount of curry powder that you personally would like for the spice level that you prefer. Toss lightly then set aside. On a serving plate Place kale greens then tomatoes and mango on top. Then put your cucumber mixture on top and sprinkle with slivered almonds.

13. Greek Cucumber Salad

Servings: 2

Ingredients:

- one English cucumber, spiralized
- one tablespoon of red onion thinly sliced
- ten black olives pitted
- half a fresh lemon
- half a cup of feta cheese crumbled
- one tablespoon of fresh oregano leaves minced
- half a cup of cherry tomatoes halved
- one red bell pepper thinly sliced
- half a tablespoon of extra virgin olive oil
- sea salt
- fresh ground pepper to taste

Directions:

Using a spiral slicer or a julienne peeler spiralize your cucumber to about the size of fettuccine size noodles. Put your cucumber spirals into a large bowl. Add bell pepper, olives, tomatoes, red onion. Squeeze over it the juice of half a lemon. Drizzle with half of the oil. Add the oregano. Toss salad gently until it is evenly coated. Add to a serving plate. Top with feta then drizzle the remaining oil over it and serve.

14. Salad of Many Colors

Servings: 4

Ingredients:

- two English cucumbers, spiralized
- one large beet, spiralized
- two carrots, spiralized
- one mango, julienned
- two tablespoons of salad dressing of your choice
  I would suggest a nice garlic dressing

Homemade Garlic-Basil Dressing Ingredients:

- one third cup of extra virgin olive oil
- one quarter cup of fresh lime juice
- one quarter cup of fresh basil finely chopped
- one tablespoon of honey
- one teaspoon of garlic
- half a teaspoon of sea salt
- one quarter teaspoon of fresh ground pepper

Directions:

Spiralize your carrots, beet, and cucumber into spaghetti size noodles. Toss with mango and dressing until all is well coated. Let it sit for a few minutes to settle then put into serving bowls and enjoy this yummy dish!

Chapter 4:

Spiralized Poultry Main Dishes

You will find a wind array of main spiral slicer dishes that you and your family will be able to enjoy for many years to come eating your way to health and wellness with these tasty recipes!

Spiralized Poultry Recipes

15. Lemon-Garlic Turkey with Zucchini Noodles

Servings: 4

Ingredients:

- half a pound of turkey breast cut into strips
- half a teaspoon of extra virgin olive oil
- two zucchini, spiralized
- two tablespoons of organic butter
- one tablespoon of parsley, minced
- zest from half a fresh lemon
- one teaspoon of minced garlic
- half a teaspoon of sea salt
- one quarter teaspoon of ground black pepper
- one quarter cup of fresh parsley chopped

Directions:

Mix together in a bowl garlic, oil, parsley, salt,

pepper, lemon juice. Add your turkey strips to the bowl and cover and marinate for 30 minutes. Spiralize your zucchini into spaghetti size noodles and set aside. In a skillet heat butter over low heat. Remove your turkey strips from marinade and reserve the marinade. Add your turkey strips to pan and cook for 4 minutes on each side or until they are cooked through and slightly browned on the outside. Add your marinade to the pan and simmer for a few minutes. Add salt and pepper to taste and remove from heat. Put on to serving plates then sprinkle with fresh parsley.

16. Mediterranean Chicken with Artichoke Hearts

Servings: 4

Ingredients:

- four chicken cutlets
- one tablespoon of extra virgin olive oil
- four tablespoons of organic butter
- one tablespoon of coconut flour
- three quarter teaspoon of basil
- half a cup of low-sodium chicken broth
- half a cup of white wine
- one quarter teaspoon of allspice
- one cup of marinated artichoke hearts drained
- eight Greek olives pitted and halved
- two tablespoons of pine nuts
- cayenne pepper sauce to desired level of spicy

Directions:

Heat a large skillet over medium heat with olive oil.
Add chicken cutlets and cook for four minutes per side

or until your chicken is browned and cooked through. Transfer you chicken to a plate and set aside. In the pan with the drippings add butter heating until melted. Add the chicken broth, wine, and a few drops of cayenne pepper sauce to desired level of spicy. Blend in the allspice, basil, and flour keep stirring until well blended. Spiralize your zucchini into fettuccine size noodles then add them to the sauce cooking for about three minutes stir gently. Remove noodles from pan. Add your artichoke hearts to the pan mixing in sauce, adding chicken cutlets back into the pan. Toss and combine them with the sauce. Remove them from heat serve over bed of zucchini noodles then top with pine nuts.

17. Spicy Chicken & Peanut Sauce with Summer Squash Noodles

Servings: 6

Ingredients:

- three summer squash, spiralized
- one quarter cup of fresh cilantro
- two zucchini, spiralized
- one teaspoon of minced garlic
- one tablespoon of low-sodium soy sauce
- half a cup of peanut butter creamy
- four tablespoons of apple cider vinegar
- two teaspoons of extra virgin olive oil
- half a teaspoon of Stevia
- five cups of diced chicken breast cooked
- two tablespoons of sesame seeds

Directions:

In a bowl add soy sauce, vinegar, peanut butter, garlic, Stevia, oil and mix until ingredients are well blended. Slowly add about one third cup of water or as much as needed to reach the desired consistency.

Spiralize your zucchini, and your summer squash into spaghetti size noodles. Boil zucchini and summer squash for three minutes then drain once vegetables have cooled. Place on serving plate top with chicken mixture then add cilantro and sesame seeds.

18. Turkey Sausage and Rutabaga Noodles

Servings: 4

Ingredients:

- three rutabaga, spiralized
- one tablespoon of organic butter
- three tablespoons of extra virgin olive oil divided
- two small red onions thinly sliced
- four tablespoons of balsamic vinegar
- pinch of sea salt
- ground pepper to taste
- four cooked turkey sausages
- two cups of spinach fresh chopped

Directions:

In a skillet heat butter with one tablespoon of oil over medium heat. Add the onions and saute for 20 minutes or until soft and golden brown. Add the spinach and saute until it is wilted. Add balsamic vinegar, increase the heat to medium-high cooking for two minutes or until the liquid is absorbed. Season with salt and pepper.

Spiralize rutabagas into spaghetti size noodles. In another pan heat in remaining two tablespoons of oil over medium heat. On one side of your skillet cook rutabaga then add turkey sausage on the other side cook sausage for five minutes or until well browned. Serve your sausage bedside your rutabaga noodles and pour spinach mixture over.

19. Spiralized Russet Potatoes & Chicken

Servings: 4

Ingredients:

- six tablespoons of organic butter, divided
- four tablespoons of sour cream
- one tablespoon of extra virgin olive oil
- one celery stalk, finely diced
- two cups of low-sodium chicken broth
- four tablespoons of coconut flour
- two tablespoons of paprika
- two white onions, thinly sliced
- one whole chicken, quartered
- four russet potatoes, spiralized

Directions:

In a dutch oven melt three tablespoons of butter on medium-low heat. Stir in the onions and saute them for 15 minutes then remove onions from the pan. Add the remaining three tablespoons of butter and melt in the Dutch oven. Add the chicken. Brown the chicken in the butter turn the chicken often. Add the chicken broth. sauteed onions, and diced celery to the chicken. Cover and simmer for one hour or until the chicken is fully cooked. Spiralize your potatoes make them into egg noodles size. In a skillet heat oil over medium heat then add the noodles and cook for eight minutes. Add your noodles to a serving plate. Remove your chicken from the Dutch oven and place on plate on top of bed of noodles. Add sour cream and flour to the gravy in the pan then pour this over your meal.

20. Chicken & Wine-Mushroom Sauce with Zucchini Noodles

Servings: 4

Ingredients:

- four zucchini, spiralized
- four tablespoons of organic butter
- two chicken breasts boneless, skinless
- one tablespoon of sea salt
- one tablespoon of black pepper
- one teaspoon of garlic minced
- half a cup of finely chopped red onion
- one cup of sliced mushrooms
- half a cup of white wine vinegar
- one third cup of half-and-half cream
- half a cup of almond flour
- chopped fresh parsley for garnish

Directions:

Spiralize your zucchini into spaghetti size noodles pat them dry with a piece of paper towel and set aside. In pan saute half of the butter over medium heat add chicken sprinkle with salt and pepper and cook until the chicken is lightly browned. Remove chicken from pan and cube into small pieces about one inch big. To the pan and drippings add the onion, garlic, mushrooms, thyme, white wine vinegar, half-and-half, flour, stir and simmer for five minutes. Mix the noodles with chicken and sauce then add to a casserole dish and bake for 30 minutes.

Chapter 5:

Spiralized Beef Main Dishes

In this chapter you will find some great tasty
spiralized beef dishes that your whole family will enjoy
and be asking you to make them not because they are
healthy but because they taste so yummy!

21.Kale & Turkey Sausage Eggplant Zucchini Lasagna

Servings: 4

Ingredients:

- two eggplant, peeled and cut into lengthwise slices of eight
- two zucchini, cut lengthwise into six slices
- one quarter cup of coconut oil melted
- four tablespoons of extra virgin olive oil
- sea salt
- fresh ground black pepper
- one teaspoon of garlic
- one onion chopped
- one teaspoon of dried Italian seasoning
- twelve ounces of ground turkey
- one five ounce pack of cheese and garlic croutons, crushed
- two cups of shredded mozzarella cheese
- one egg lightly beaten

- half a cup of grated Parmesan cheese
- one fifteen ounce container of ricotta cheese
- one quarter cup of fresh basil, chopped
- one chunky can of pasta sauce

Directions:

Heat the oven to 425 degrees Fahrenheit. Coat two 15×10×1 inch baking pans with cooking spray. Use a Mandoline slicer to cut the eggplant and zucchini for even slices. Arrange your eggplant and zucchini on the baking sheets. Brush the tops with one quarter cup of olive oil. Season with salt and pepper. Bake for 15 minutes or until tender. Remove from oven. Reduce the temperature to 375 degrees Fahrenheit. In a large skillet heat one tablespoon of coconut oil over medium heat add the ground turkey and cook for eight minutes until it is browned. Add onion and garlic and cook for another five minutes. Stir in the pasta sauce, Italian seasoning, and three tablespoons of basil.

Remove from heat. In bowl mix ricotta cheese, egg, and parmesan cheese until well blended. Coat a 13×9 inch baking dish with cooking spray. Layer half of the eggplant into it. Top eggplant with ricotta mixture, half of the zucchini, and one and a half cups of pasta sauce and one cup of mozzarella. Top with the remaining zucchini, pasta, eggplant and ricotta mixture. Bake for 35 minutes or until hot and cheese is bubbling. Remove from oven. In a small bowl mix crushed croutons with remaining two tablespoons of melted coconut oil. Sprinkle evenly over the top then add the remaining one cup of Mozzarella cheese. Bake for another ten minutes until cheese is melted and croutons are slightly toasted. Remove from oven and let stand for five minutes. Sprinkle with remaining one tablespoon of basil and enjoy!

22. Curried Beef with Sweet Potato Noodles

Servings: 6

Ingredients:

- three tablespoons of coconut oil, melted
- one pound of beef stew, cut into one inch pieces
- pinch of sea salt
- fresh ground pepper to taste
- one large white onion, sliced
- one teaspoon of garlic minced
- one cinnamon stick
- one bay leaf
- two medium tomatoes, quartered
- three tablespoons of chutney
- two zucchini, spiralized
- two yellow squash, spiralized
- three quarter cups of milk
- one quarter teaspoon of dried red pepper
- one teaspoon of fresh lemon juice
- one tablespoon of curry powder

- one tablespoon of ginger minced
- two tablespoons of fresh cilantro, chopped

Directions:

In a large skillet on medium heat, heat one tablespoon of oil. Add your beef in batches as it makes for easier browning. Season beef with salt and pepper. Sear your beef for about six minutes or until brown on all sides. Add more oil if necessary. With a slotted spoon transfer your beef to a plate. Heat the remaining oil in the same skillet adding onions saute for about five minutes then return the beef to the skillet. Add cinnamon stick, bay leaf, red pepper, garlic and stir. Mix in the milk, tomatoes, lemon juice, ginger, curry powder, and some salt and bring to a boil. Reduce heat to simmer and cover stir occasionally for two hours or until beef is tender. Remove the cover and increase the heat until the juices start to thicken. Spiralize yellow squash, and zucchini into spaghetti size noodles. Add your noodles to the beef mixture and toss gently cooking for another three minutes. Top with cilantro and serve.

23. Turkey Spaghetti Sauce & Zucchini Noodles

Servings: 4

Ingredients:

- one pound of ground turkey
- one yellow onion diced
- one tablespoon of garlic minced
- 28 ounce can of crushed tomatoes
- half a teaspoon of dried oregano
- one teaspoon of dried basil
- 1-26 ounce can of pasta sauce
- two zucchini, spiralized
- two tablespoons of coconut oil, melted
- Parmesan cheese

Directions:

In a large saucepan saute ground turkey over medium heat for ten minutes or until it is browned. Add onions and one tablespoon of oil, saute onion for five minutes. Add garlic, pasta sauce, tomatoes, oregano, and basil, bring to a boil. Lower to a simmer and cover for 45 minutes. Use a spiral slicer to spiralize your zucchini into spaghetti size noodles. In a different pan add remaining oil and saute the zucchini for about five minutes. Put zucchini noodles on serving plates then top with sauce and garnish with Parmesan then serve.

24. Garlic Pork Chops & Applesauce with Zucchini Noodles

Servings: 2

Ingredients:

- two zucchini, spiralized
- two pork chops
- one serving of unsweetened applesauce
- dash of cinnamon
- 1-28 ounce can of diced tomatoes, drained
- four tablespoons of balsamic dressing
- two tablespoons of fresh basil, chopped
- black pepper to taste
- garlic powder
- one teaspoon of minced garlic
- fresh parsley, chopped for garnish

Directions:

Heat oven to 375 degrees Fahrenheit. Spray a baking sheet place your pork chops on baking sheet and sprinkle with garlic powder lightly on both sides. Bake for 20 minutes then flip over and bake for another 20 minutes or until both sides are golden brown. Add a tablespoon or so of applesauce on top of pork chops in the last five minutes of baking and add sprinkle of cinnamon. Put bake into oven to finish baking. Spiralize your zucchini into spaghetti size noodles. In a small pan put tomatoes, minced garlic, basil, and balsamic dressing. Put up to medium-low heat and add zucchini noodles and stir lightly cooking for another five minutes. Take pork chops and put on serving plates and add the zucchini noodles on the side garnish with parsley and enjoy!

25. Alfredo Pasta with Asparagus & Mushrooms

Servings: 2

Ingredients:

- two zucchini, spiralized
- two tablespoons of extra virgin olive oil
- five ounces of sliced mushrooms
- half a cup of red bell pepper, thinly sliced
- one cup of asparagus, chopped
- one bottle of store bought Alfredo sauce
- add black pepper to taste
- two ounces of prosciutto, chopped

Directions:

Spiralize your zucchini into spaghetti size noodles. Set aside. In a frying pan add the oil, asparagus, mushrooms, and prosciutto. Saute until the prosciutto is lightly crispy. Add in the Alfredo sauce and zucchini and toss lightly on simmer for about three minutes. Remove from heat. Serve in pasta bowls and garnish with fresh parsley or basil.

26. Garlic Pork & Zucchini Noodles

Servings: 4

Ingredients:

- one pound of ground pork
- one small red onion, diced
- one red bell pepper, diced
- one teaspoon of garlic, minced
- pinch of black pepper
- pinch of sea salt
- 14 ounce can of coconut milk
- one carrot, spiralized
- two zucchini, spiralized
- half a cup of almond butter
- one quarter cup of low-sodium soy sauce
- two tablespoons of lime juice
- two tablespoons of sriracha

Directions:

Spiralize your carrot, and zucchini into spaghetti size noodles. Set these aside in bowl lined with paper towel. In a frying pan add oil on medium heat and pork, onion, bell pepper, garlic, and salt and pepper. Saute for seven minutes or so or until pork is no longer pink in color. Toss in carrot and cook for another three minutes. Toss in zucchini and cook for another two minutes. Remove from heat and place into serving bowls. In a small saucepan whisk together milk, soy sauce, butter, lime juice, and sriracha cook on low heat for several minutes. Pour the sauce over the noodles and pork in bowls. Sprinkle with chopped cilantro as a garnish.

27. Potato Spaghetti Pie

Servings: 4

Ingredients:

- one sweet potato, spiralized
- two russet potatoes, spiralized
- one tablespoon of organic butter melted
- one egg beaten
- cooking spray
- one quarter cup of Parmesan, grated
- two tablespoons of coconut oil, melted
- half a red onion, chopped
- one teaspoon garlic, minced
- one cup of low-fat cottage cheese, drained
- half a cup of mozzarella cheese, shredded
- eight ounces of ground Italian sausage
- one eight ounce can of tomato sauce
- one teaspoon of dried oregano

Directions:

Preheat oven to 350 degrees Fahrenheit. Spiralize your potatoes into spaghetti size noodles. Stir in butter, egg, and Parmesan. Coat a nine inch pie plate with cooking spray. Then, take the potato mixture and press it onto the bottom and sides of the pie plate to form a crust. In a skillet heat oil over medium heat adding sausage, onion, bell pepper, and garlic cooking for several minutes. Drain. Stir in tomato sauce and oregano and heat through. Spread the cottage cheese over the top of the potato pie crust. Spread meat mixture over cottage cheese then top with shredded mozzarella. Bake for 25 minutes or until it is baked through. Let it cool for five minutes then serve.

Chapter 6:

Spiralized Fish & Seafood Main Dishes

Something that my family loves is seafood so if you and your family love them too you will enjoy these wonderful spiralized fish and seafood dishes offered in this chapter. This food group is great source of omega-3's also known as brain food!

28. Lime-Garlic Shrimp with Spinach & Zucchini Noodles

Serves: 2 (just double up on ingredients to make enough for 4 servings)

Ingredients:

- 15 large shrimp, peeled and deveined
- two zucchini, spiralized
- half a teaspoon of coconut oil, melted
- one tablespoon of fresh parsley, minced
- zest from half a lime
- lime juice from half a lime
- one tablespoon of organic butter
- one cup of baby spinach
- sea salt
- black pepper

Directions:

In a bowl combine oil, garlic, lime juice, lime zest, salt and pepper. Let sit for 30 minutes. Spiralize your zucchini into spaghetti size noodles. Set aside. Heat up butter over medium heat. Add shrimp with marinade. Cook for 30 seconds. Remove shrimp with slotted spoon from pan and set aside. Add your zucchini noodles to the pan and toss lightly for two minutes. Add spinach, shrimp to pan with zucchini. Add salt and pepper to taste and squeeze juice from remaining half of lime into it.

29. Shrimp & Scallops with Butternut Squash

Serves: 6

Ingredients:

- two large butternut squash necks, spiralized
- four tablespoons of coconut oil, melted
- one pound of jumbo shrimp, peeled, and deveined
- one pound of scallops
- one tablespoon of garlic, minced
- one red onion, chopped
- 28- ounce can of diced tomatoes
- quarter teaspoon of paprika
- three turkey sausage, thickly sliced
- one teaspoon of black pepper
- half a cup of low-sodium chicken broth
- six tablespoons of fresh parsley, chopped
- lime wedges for garnish (optional)

Directions:

Spiralize your butternut squash into spaghetti size noodles. Set aside. In skillet heat three tablespoons of oil and add shrimp on medium heat. Cook for five minutes turn once. Transfer shrimp to a plate. Add scallops to skillet and sear for half a minute on each side. Transfer to plate with shrimp. Add turkey sausage slices to the pan cook for three minutes. Add remaining one tablespoon of oil, garlic, tomatoes, salt, paprika, pepper, saute for several minutes. Add chicken broth to skillet reduce the heat to medium. Stir in the squash noodles and simmer for several minutes. Add shrimp and scallops to the mixture in skillet. Add to serving dish and garnish with fresh parsley. Serve and enjoy!

30. Tuna & Zucchini Casserole

Serves: 4

Ingredients:

- two zucchini, spiralize one zucchini, and cut the other into one quarter- inch slices
- one celery stalk, chopped
- one teaspoon of garlic, minced
- two teaspoons of extra virgin olive oil, divided
- 2- 5 ounce cans of tuna, drained and flaked
- half a cup of mayonnaise
- half a cup of low-fat sour cream
- two tablespoons of Dijon mustard
- half a teaspoon of dried Thyme
- one quarter teaspoon of black pepper
- one cup of Monterey Jack cheese, shredded
- two tablespoons of fresh basil, chopped
- three green onions, thinly sliced

Directions:

Preheat oven to 375 degrees Fahrenheit. Spiralize one zucchini into spaghetti size noodles set in paper towel lined bowel. Set aside. In a large skillet saute zucchini slices in a teaspoon of oil until crispy. Remove from skillet. Saute celery in the remaining oil until crispy. Add garlic and saute for a minute or so. In large bowl add tuna, sour cream, green onions, thyme, salt, pepper, mayonnaise, and mustard and celery. Mix well. Add spiralized zucchini and toss to combine. In a greased 11×7 baking dish; add half of zucchini noodle mixture. Then, top with zucchini slices and repeat layers. Cook at 375 degrees Fahrenheit for 30 minutes. Sprinkle basil over to of casserole and serve.

31. Salmon & Creamy Dill Sauce with Zucchini Noodles

Serves: 4

Ingredients:

- two zucchini, spiralized
- one pound of fresh salmon, cut into four evenly sized pieces
- pinch of sea salt
- pinch of black pepper
- one serving cup of Greek plain yogurt
- one tablespoon of fresh dill weed
- half a teaspoon of grated lemon zest
- one tablespoon of lemon juice
- one tablespoon of coconut oil, melted

Directions:

Preheat oven 375 degrees Fahrenheit. Place your salmon in a large baking dish with the skin side facing down. Brush with olive oil over salmon. Season with salt and pepper. Bake for 25 minutes. Spiralize zucchini into fettuccine size noodles. When the salmon is almost done place your noodles in the boiling water for two minutes then remove. In skillet add oil on medium heat add the zucchini noodles and saute for a few minutes or until noodles become tender. In bowl mix yogurt, dill, lemon zest, lemon juice, and pepper. Mix well. Place zucchini noodles onto serving plate then add some dill sauce. Add your salmon on top and add more dill sauce on top of salmon.

32. Tilapia & Dijon Cream Sauce with Pasta

Serves: 2

Ingredients:

- two tilapia filets
- two zucchini, spiralized
- pinch of sea salt
- one lime, halved
- three quarter of a cup of low-sodium chicken broth
- three tablespoons of Dijon mustard
- one teaspoon of cilantro
- two tablespoons of light whipping cream
- one teaspoon of ground cumin

Directions:

Preheat the oven to 375 degrees Fahrenheit. Spiralize your zucchini into fettuccine size noodles. Set into bowl lined with paper towel and set aside. Spray a baking sheet with cooking spray then place your tilapia fillets on it. Lightly squeeze some fresh squeezed lime juice over your filets. Season with salt and pepper. Bake fish for 15 minutes or until it is cooked through.

In a frying pan add cilantro, mustard, chicken broth, and cumin. Whisk these ingredients around mixing them well, add your zucchini noodles and whipping cream simmer for two minutes or until heated through. Remove your zucchini noodles leaving sauce still in the pan with utensil that is porous. Transfer the noodles to serving plates. Top with the tilapia, and pour cream sauce over the top and serve.

33. Spicy Shrimp & Parsnip Noodles

Serves: 4

Ingredients:

- one pound of shrimp, peeled, and deveined
- three parsnips, spiralized
- one tablespoon of fresh parsley, chopped
- sea salt and pepper to taste
- half a teaspoon of chili powder
- one teaspoon of garlic, minced
- one quarter of a teaspoon of red pepper flakes
- half a cup of low-sodium chicken broth
- three tablespoons of coconut oil, melted
- one cup of red onion, diced

Directions:

Spiralize your parsnips into wide egg noodle style noodles. Set aside in a bowl lined with paper towel. In a skillet heat to medium heat two tablespoons of coconut oil, add onion and saute for five minutes. Add the garlic and the red pepper flakes sauteing for an additional two minutes. Add the remaining one tablespoon of oil to skillet along with your parsnip noodles. Add salt, pepper, chili powder.

Cook for five minutes or until your noodles are softened. Move your noodles to the side of your skillet then add the chicken broth and shrimp. Cook the shrimp for two minutes then turn shrimp over to cook the other side for two more minutes. Gently toss the shrimp and noodles together. Remove from heat and put into serving bowls add fresh parsley as a garnish if you wish and enjoy!

34. Crab & Kohlrabi Noodles

Serves: 4

Ingredients:

- two kohlrabi, spiralized
- one large package of frozen crab pieces
- two tablespoons of organic butter
- two tablespoons of coconut oil, melted
- half a cup of dry white wine
- two tablespoons of lemon juice
- half a cup of fresh parsley, chopped
- sea salt
- black pepper, freshly ground
- Parmesan cheese, shredded
- one cup of asparagus, cut diagonally into three inch pieces

Directions:

Allow your package of crab meat to defrost. Once crab meat is defrosted slice it up into smaller pieces or shred. Spiralize your kohlrabi into spaghetti size noodles. Put your noodles into a bowl lined with paper towel and set aside. In a skillet heat up your butter and oil over medium heat. Add the garlic and saute. Add lemon juice and wine and simmer for ten minutes. Add the asparagus and your kohlrabi noodles cover the skillet for five minutes to steam. Allow asparagus to become tender-crisp and your kohlrabi soft. Add your pieces of crab meat and toss lightly. Add salt and pepper, top with parsley and parmesan once in serving bowls.

35. Grilled Shrimp & Lime Basil Dressing with Zucchini Noodles

Serves: 4

Ingredients:

- one shallot, chopped
- one tablespoon of red wine vinegar
- one teaspoon of garlic, minced
- two cups of fresh basil, chopped
- one third cup of slivered almonds, divided
- half a cup of coconut oil, melted
- one tablespoon of extra virgin olive oil
- one pound of shrimp, peeled and deveined
- three zucchini, spiralized
- salt and pepper to taste
- four tablespoons of lemon basil dressing

Directions:

In a blender combine lime zest, half of your almonds, basil, shallot, garlic, red pepper flakes, extra virgin olive oil, and red wine vinegar. Blend until these ingredients are smooth. Season with salt and pepper then set aside. Heat a tablespoon of coconut oil over medium heat adding shrimp. Cook your shrimp for four minutes or until fully cooked. Remove shrimp from heat. Mix in two tablespoons of lemon basil dressing. Transfer your shrimp to a serving bowl using slotted spoon and set aside. Spiralize zucchini into spaghetti size noodles add them to the same pan you used for your shrimp and saute noodles for two minutes. Add two remaining tablespoons of lemon basil dressing toss to coat then remove from heat. Place noodles on serving dishes then put the shrimp on top of noodles season with salt, fresh ground pepper and remaining slivered almonds. Enjoy!

Chapter 7:

Spiralized Vegetarian Main Dishes

Here are some great tasting spiralized vegetarian recipes that you and your family are sure to enjoy. It is a healthy way to cut back on meats or if you are just trying to add a different approach to the family meal. It can be fun and exciting getting away from the regular meals and serving your family a new dish that is healthy, quick and easy to prepare.

36. Sauteed Mushrooms & Baby Spinach with Squash Noodles

Serves: 4

Ingredients:

- two sweet potato squash, spiralized
- five ounces of mushrooms, sliced
- eight ounces of baby spinach
- half a cup of low-sodium chicken broth
- one teaspoon of garlic, minced
- one leek, thinly sliced
- four tablespoons of coconut oil, melted
- half a cup of dry white wine
- salt and pepper
- two green onions, chopped
- two tablespoons of fresh parsley, chopped

Directions:

Spiralize your sweet potato squash into spaghetti size noodles. Place in a bowl lined with paper towel and set aside. In a frying pan saute your leek and garlic for two minutes in oil. Add mushrooms and continue to saute until mushrooms become browned. Add your spinach to the pan and pour in the chicken broth and wine. Add salt and pepper. Stir in your noodles and saute for a few more minutes tossing lightly. Remove from heat and serve right away.

37. Butternut Squash & Roasted Sweet Potato with Zucchini Pasta

Serves: 4

Ingredients:

- one butternut squash, peeled
- two sweet potatoes, spiralized
- two zucchini, spiralized
- one cup of asparagus, cut into three inch lengths
- half a cup of Monterey Jack cheese
- one third cup of dry white wine
- sea salt and pepper to taste

Directions:

Preheat your oven to 375 degrees Fahrenheit. Spiralize your zucchini into spaghetti size noodles. Put into a bowl lined with paper towel and set aside. Spiralize your sweet potato and neck of butternut squash into spaghetti size noodles. Remove the seeds from the bulb of your squash and chop into cubes about an inch in size. Place your asparagus and butternut cubes on a baking sheet and drizzle with oil tossing to coat. Sprinkle with salt and pepper. Roast for 25 minutes or until they are tender and crispy. In a skillet add two tablespoons of coconut oil over medium heat adding sweet potato and squash noodles. Saute your noodles for about four minutes or until they are beginning to soften. Add the cheese, wine, and zucchini noodles into pan and toss to coat. Cook for about another two minutes or until the cheese has melted. Remove from heat. Add your roasted butternut squash and asparagus to the top of noodles after they have been put on serving plates and enjoy!

38. Anchovies & Roasted Garlic Tomatoes with Butternut Squash Noodles

Serves: 4

Ingredients:

- two anchovy fillets packed in oil
- one quarter cup of organic butter
- one teaspoon of garlic, minced
- 1-28- ounce can of crushed tomatoes
- one butternut squash, spiralized
- Parmesan cheese, finely grated for garnish
- freshly ground black pepper
- sea salt
- half a teaspoon of red pepper flakes
- half a cup of white onion, finely sliced
- half cup of vegetable broth

Directions:

Preheat oven to 375 degrees Fahrenheit. Combine tomatoes, anchovies, garlic, butter, red pepper flakes on a

13×9 inch baking sheet. Season with salt and pepper.
Roast this tomato mix in the oven for 40 minutes. Gently
toss the mixture halfway through the cooking process.
Add the mixture and vegetable broth to large sauce pan.
Spiralize your butternut squash into fettuccine size
noodles then add to pan with tomato sauce mixture.
Cook over medium heat for seven minutes. Top with
Parmesan cheese and serve.

39. Butternut Squash & Rosemary Sauce with Zucchini Noodles

Servings: 4

Ingredients:

- one butternut squash
- one tablespoon of garlic, minced
- one cup of half-and-half whipping cream
- pinch of dried rosemary
- three tablespoons of coconut oil, melted, divided
- one white onion, chopped
- half a cup of low-sodium chicken broth
- fourteen ounces of portabella mushrooms, sliced
- two green onions, chopped
- four zucchini, spiralized
- fresh ground black pepper
- sea salt to taste

Directions:

Preheat oven to 425 degrees Fahrenheit. Slice your butternut squash in half lengthwise and remove the seeds.

Place the cut side down of squash onto the baking sheet and cover with tin foil. Roast squash for about 45 minutes or until the squash is tender. Cool squash. When your squash has cooled scoop out and add to blender. In a small pan heat one tablespoon of coconut oil over medium heat. Add onions and garlic and saute for three minutes.

Add the onions, garlic, rosemary, chicken broth, whipping cream to the blender with the squash. Blend until smooth. Add the remaining coconut oil to large pan and saute the mushrooms for about five minutes. Spiralize your zucchini into fettuccine size noodles. Add these noodles to the mushrooms and saute for three minutes. Add the sauce to the pan and continue to cook for another three minutes or until sauce is hot. Put into serving bowls and garnish with chopped green onions and black pepper.

40. Avocado, Carrot, Feta Wrap with Zucchini Noodles

Servings: for 1 Wrap

Ingredients:

- three tablespoons of feta cheese, crumbled
- two tablespoons of hummus
- one tortilla whole wheat wrap
- one small carrot, spiralized
- half a zucchini, spiralized
- one quarter cup of chick peas, drained and rinsed
- one quarter avocado, sliced
- fresh ground black pepper to taste

Directions:

Take your tortilla and spread the hummus evenly over it. Add avocado. Season with pepper. Spiralize carrot, and zucchini into spaghetti size noodles. Place carrots and zucchini noodles into wrap cover with chick peas. Add feta cheese to top. Roll up and secure with toothpicks. You can make two smaller wraps by slicing it in half. This makes a great meal when you are on the go and need something healthy and quick!

Conclusion

I hope that you and your family will enjoy making these healthy fun, spiralized recipes for many years to come. It can be very challenging in the world today to try and find foods that your whole family will enjoy. Sometimes when you approach the way you present foods to them by using spiralizing them for example it can truly draw their attention to the meals being put in front of them in a new refreshed outlook. Healthy foods do not have to be boring the recipes in this book will most certainly prove that! Best of luck to cooking your way to a life full of optimal health and wellness!

Finally, if you enjoyed this book, then I'd like to ask you for a big favor, would you be kind enough to leave a review for this book on Amazon? It'd be greatly appreciated!

Book 3
Sugar Detox:
Beat Sugar Cravings and Overcome Sugar Addiction to Lose Weight and Increase Energy in 21 Days!

Introduction

Beat Sugar Cravings and Overcome Sugar Addiction!

You have certainly made a step in the right direction in deciding to download this book, it will help guide you towards a healthier lifestyle through the information that it offers you. It is so important in life that you take time to take care of yourself and your loved ones. In this fast paced world we live in we often find ourselves choosing fast foods that offer us little to no nutritional value, but instead contribute to the weight gain we want to get rid of. When reading this book you are going to learn how to make your life a healthier one by using the 21 day sugar detox diet.

Making changes for the most part is never easy, but when you know in your heart you are making changes that are going to improve your lifestyle then they will be well worth any sacrifices you may have to make. You may have a sugar addiction that you are worried has become out of control, perhaps diabetes runs in your family and you are concerned that if you do not make serious changes in your eating habits you too may end up with diabetes or even a worse health condition such as heart disease. Whatever the reasons are behind you deciding that you wanted to take a closer look into sugar detox you will find the information collected in this book to be very informative covering many aspects on the topic of sugar such as how it affects our bodies. You will be given some sugar-free recipes that you can try out along with a bonus seven day sugar detox meal planner to help start you on your way to a healthier lifestyle.

Once you have completed the 21 day sugar detox diet you will be guided in how to introduce sugar back into your lifestyle, making sure that you are choosing good sugars over bad. Knowing the bad sugars and what to look out for will make your challenge a more successful one. That is why I am starting this book at the beginning with what and where sugar comes from. Through each chapter we will go through a new experience, each one connected to sugar in one way or another. You are going to have a whole new start once you have gotten rid of the sugar toxins in your body that cause you to have horrible sugar cravings. When you have gone through the sugar detox process you are going to start afresh. With a whole new approach to what kinds of sugars you are going to have as part of your diet and the ones that you have decided no longer are fit into your new healthy lifestyle you are not only going to look great but you are going to feel great! Your body is going to thank you in a way that it knows how to by making you feel more happy, energized, and full of life than you have in a very long time! I wish you great success in your 21 day sugar detox—I know your body is going to be thanking you for it that's for sure! What better way to show some self-love by giving your body a much needed sugar detox!

Chapter 1:

What is Sugar?

What is sugar?

Most of us know it by its general name 'Sugar' not as its full name 'short-chain, soluble carbohydrates.' Most of us are well aware of these sweet tasting carbohydrates that make our taste buds tingle, made from a combination of oxygen, carbon, and hydrogen.

Sugar is what I call the sweet tasting poison—due to the many health problems that are associated with it. In order to understand sugar better we must learn where it comes from and how it is made.

How is sugar made?

Sugar is grown by sugar farmers who grow it in the

form of sugar beet plants, and sugar cane. Once the farmers have harvested the sugar it is processed using wash and dry cycles that extract and refine the sugar juice into fine crystals. These crystals are sold as unbleached, they have a higher content of molasses this is known as raw sugar. Table sugar is more refined lowering the content of molasses crystals this is sold as bleached sugar.

How does our bodies use sugar?

The key source of energy for our bodies is glucose, this is a simple sugar. Glucose is the primary source of energy for our brains. If we are lacking in glucose this could impair psychological processes that require mental effort to complete. When we are doing our daily work it is glucose that keeps us functioning, helping our muscles work at their best when doing strenuous work for example.

The red blood cells in our bodies use glucose as a source of energy. Glucose is also important during pregnancy helping to produce milk, and form cells. The body will take extra glucose and store it in the form of glycogen. In the liver there is a process called glycogenesis that makes glycogen chains up to thousands of glucose molecules long. The body will break down parts of these chains when it needs to use them for energy when there is no primary sources available. This process can happen during workouts, sleep, meals, to prevent dangerous drops occurring in a person's blood sugar.

Without sugar the human body is unable to function. Now you are wondering why sugar gets a bad wrap if we need it to survive. This has to do with knowing the difference between good and bad sugars. Simple sugars lack in nutritional value.

Differences between simple and complex carbohydrates.

All carbohydrates have units of sugar in them. Carbohydrates are found in all foods except for animal protein, and fats or oils. What makes them different from one another is the amounts of sugar units that they contain.

Three subcategories of Carbohydrates:

1. Simple Carbohydrates (simple sugars)
2. Complex Carbohydrates (starches)

3. Dietary fiber

Bad carbohydrates.

The bad carbohydrates are made up of one or two units of sugar. Because of their simple structure the body is able to break them down and digest them quickly, this does not offer proper nutrients, and energy that the body requires. Simple carbohydrates are quickly released into the bloodstream causing a spike in the body's energy level soon to be followed by a crash in energy.

Foods that are filled with these empty calories are well known to most of us some examples being: cakes, cookies, chips, soft drinks, white, rice, and white bread. Sucrose, fructose, lactose are also forms of simple sugars. You should try and avoid these as they offer no nutritional value.

Good carbohydrates.

Complex carbohydrates are the good carbohydrates, these contain more than two units of sugar linked together. With complex carbohydrates they can have anywhere from three to millions of units of sugar linked together. Due to their complexity the body takes longer to digest them before it releases them into the blood stream in a more slow fashion and evenly than simple carbohydrates.

Dietary fiber.

Dietary fiber is another kind of complex carbohydrate. It does not offer a source of energy, but it provides the body with other positive benefits. Fiber is classed as either insoluble fiber or soluble fiber. This is based on whether or not it dissolves in water. The digestive enzymes of the human body are incapable of breaking down either types of fibers. This is why fibers do not add additional calories to your diet and cannot be converted into glucose. Because fiber can't be digested by the human body it is valuable. Insoluble fiber is a natural laxative. You can find it in foods such as: whole grains, whole wheat, beets, beans, bran, carrots, and cabbage just to name a few. Fiber will help you to feel fuller and it will help to move solid materials through your intestinal track. It helps to prevent digestive disorders such as constipation.

Soluble fiber is found in foods such as: oats, beans, barley, fruits, rice, seeds, and seaweed helps to lower the amount of cholesterol that is in your blood. Soluble is a natural aid in helping prevent heart disease.

Not all simple sugars are bad.

First you must know that all bad sugars are simple, but know to get you really confused—not all simple sugars are considered bad. It all depends on where the sugar comes from. For example you can get simple sugars from foods such as: whole grains, nuts, beans, fruits, and vegetables, these all contain simple sugars but these foods are part of the food group known as 'whole foods.' Basically what this means is that they don't just contain sugar but also contain vitamins, minerals, and proteins. For this reason they are more than just empty calories. They are in a group that offers 'good sugars' that are natural, that are often referred to as 'natural sugars.'

That heaping teaspoon or two full of refined table sugar is the type of sugar that is considered the 'bad sugar.' This is also known as "added sugar" in the health industry, it contains no fiber or minerals it is just empty calories.

Chapter 2:
Health Issues Associated with Sugar

Effects of bad sugar on the body.

Consumption of sugar is at an all-time high and along with this it is affecting our health in a bad way. Studies have revealed that the average American consumes 156 pounds of added sugar every year! The majority of these high added sugars comes from fructose corn syrup. Soft drinks, fruit juices, and sports drinks are all loaded to the brim with added sugars. Many foods that we may not think have sugars indeed do have sugars. Processed foods such as pasta sauce in a bottle, barbeque sauce, bologna, cheese spread are all known just to name a few to have loads of sugar in them. Even baby formulas have the equivalent of one can of soda pop of sugar in them. So this is showing that are babies are becoming addicted to sugar from an early age.

Most people when they think of sugar in high intake they think of weight gain. The truth of the matter is that weight gain is only one of the many negative side effects of sugar. There is many life threatening diseases that can be caused by sugar. It can also have effects on the body that are not life threatening but do inhibit the quality of a person's life.

How does sugar cause disease?

When excessive amounts of intake of sugar are ingested into the body this leaves extra sugar molecules in the bloodstream. These sugars that are left unused in the bloodstream must go somewhere so they latch on to protein molecules throughout the entire body. They are called advanced glaciation end products these cause massive inflammation in the body as well as damaging tissue and causing premature aging. Many diseases that we normally associate with aging are caused by this process.

Normally when you have swelling or redness in an area of the body this is a sign that your body is trying to repair tissue and heal the wound. This is referred to as acute inflammation.

With Chronic inflammation the body no longer is capable of turning off the inflammatory response and it begins attacking healthy tissue mistaking it for something that may cause harm. Time magazine named inflammation "The Secret Killer" in 2004 because when it runs out of control it is causing all kinds of damage to many parts of the body. Controlling sugar intake is just one of the ways that you can help ensure that you are avoiding developing diseases due to chronic inflammation.

The following conditions can be provoked by a high sugar diet:

Weight gain.

The number of Americans that are considered over-weight has more than doubled since 1975. When you carry excess weight it increases your risk of developing, kidney disease, heart disease, and diabetes. When you are consuming sugars that are not from the "whole foods" category then you are consuming empty calories which leads to weight gain.

The body only stores 12 hours' worth of glycogen the rest of it is converted by the liver into fat.

Diabetes.

It is predicted that by the year 2050 one in three Americans will have diabetes. This grim future can be prevented if we eat better, exercise more, and lower our consumption of sugar. Diabetes is a common disease that is caused by a high sugar and high fat diet. When the pancreas fails to produce adequate insulin when the blood sugar rises Diabetes occurs. The pancreas becomes overworked and wears down and diabetes sets in. If you are over-weight and are consuming a lot of simple sugars these two factors can contribute to developing diabetes.

Heart disease.

Your body has a higher risk of developing heart disease if you are on a high sugar diet. This is especially true in women. There is no exact amount of sugar at this point that is known to make this change. It has been determined by professionals that if someone is drinking just one soft drink a day this could triple the risk of developing heart disease for some people. Since sugar is known to also contribute to high blood pressure and unhealthy cholesterol levels, it seems to me no surprise that heart disease would be following close behind as a result of a high sugar diet.

Insomnia.

Insulin is produced by the pancreas caused by the sugars, simple sugars are causing bursts of insulin to be produced by the pancreas. It can be very hard on our bodies to adjust to these highs and lows in our glucose levels. The hormone cortisol helps regulate the glucose in your body's heart, muscles, and vital organs making sure that they have enough glucose (energy) to continue doing what they need to do to help keep you alive.

Your body can become stressed out when the cortisol is increased due to highs and lows of insulin and glucose making your body start to experience things like pounding heart and sweaty palms as symptoms of stress. You can have trouble trying to sleep during these times because your body will feel like it is trying to run a fast paced race.

Lack of Focus.

Sugar can cause various mental issues. Your brain is very sensitive and it will react quickly to chemical changes in your body. Consuming glutamic acid that is found in many vegetables will help you to achieve efficient brain function. The bacteria in the intestines that manufacture vitamin B complexes begin to die when sugar is consumed. The result of declining levels of vitamin B complex is that glutamic acid is not processed and this can cause results such as short-term memory and numerical calculative abilities. It can also lead to a confused mental state, juvenile criminal behavior has also been linked to this.

Research has also discovered that sugar can cause free radicals to appear in the brain that can make it difficult to focus on both menial and complicated tasks. You could also find it hard to pay attention and listen to others.

Dental Issues.

The blood becomes very thick and sticky due to sugar content. The tiny capillaries that supply the gums and teeth with vital nutrients are inhibited by this. This can result in gum disease and teeth that are deficient of necessary nutrients.

Some other disorders that sugar plays a major role in are: depression, cataracts, Alzheimer's, disease, atherosclerosis along with many other diseases.

Chapter 3:
Dealing with Sugar Addiction

There is many nutrition experts that view the large consumption of sugars just as harmful as any other drug. When white sugar is processed it is stripped down to nothing but carbohydrates and pure calories. It contains no enzymes, vitamins, fats, minerals, or proteins. This really makes it a non-food. It is a pure chemical that is derived from plant sources that many say is purer than cocaine.

Studies have shown that the brain reacts to sugar much in the same way that it reacts to opiates like morphine, and heroine. Sugar can have a euphoric effect on the mind and body. We naturally try achieve this feeling every time we consume sugar, like all drugs it forces us to consume more and more to achieve that high. There have been studies down on humans and animals that have shown when sugar is removed suddenly from diets it would cause withdrawal symptoms similar to someone getting off narcotics.

The body has a chemical dependency on sugar that suffers when the sugar is removed and this can result in cravings, anxiety, and even the shakes in the addict.

Your body can consume two to four teaspoons of sugar a day without any problems. One can of coke contains 10.5 teaspoons of sugar. This is not including the other sugary foods that you would ingest throughout the day. Research has shown that the average person consumes twenty-six teaspoons of sugar a day. That is six to twelve times more than your body can handle.

The National Health Association recommends that the daily consumption of sugar a day for men should be 70 grams, and for women 50 grams a day.

Do you think you are addicted to sugar?

Researchers claim that most of us are addicted to sugar. You can ask yourself these questions to find out if you are indeed addicted to sugar.

When you are thinking about cutting sugar out of your diet do you worry about not eating certain specific foods anymore?

Do you find yourself eating certain foods even when you are not hungry? Do you just feel like you are craving them?

Do you overeat then find that you are tired and sluggish and need to lie down?

Do you find it hard to stop at one scoop of ice-cream?

Do you have health issues due to your diet, but you still haven't made changes to help yourself?

Do you find it very difficult to walk past a sugary treat without indulging in it even if you are not hungry?

Do you have routines that are set up around sugar?

Are there times in your day where you feel that you cannot make it through the day unless you get a sugar fix?

Do you find that you can become moody without your sugar fix?

Kicking the habit.

What is a detox? Detox is short for detoxification, it is a natural way to cleanse your body of harmful toxins that enter it through environmental pollutants or diet. If these are left in your body they can lead to adverse effects, disease and even death.

When you are doing a detox your skin, lungs, kidneys, intestines, liver and lymphatic system will all work together to turn toxins in your body into less harmful compounds that your body will be able to easily eliminate.

When you do a detox this process will remove dietary and environmental toxins from your body. There are three goals within a detox diet:

1. Increase your intake of nutrients, antioxidants, minerals, and vitamins that can help your body to repair and cleanse itself.

2. Eat mostly organic foods this will minimize the amount of chemicals going into your body.

3. Increase the amount of high fiber foods that you eat and water so that your body will be able to excrete harmful toxins.

Why should you use the sugar detox diet?

Many doctors claim that the only way that you will be able to kick sugar addiction and the curse that it has on your body is to undergo a natural process of eliminating the toxin (sugar) from your body.

Doing a sugar detox is the quickest way to effectively remove sugar from your system, break the dangerous cycle of unhealthy sugar cravings and give you a new fresh start to a healthier lifestyle. You will feel totally energized after the sugar detox, feeling great and healthier than you have in a long time!

Make sure to run the plan of doing a detox by your doctor. As long as you are not pregnant or have major issues with insulin or blood sugar, a sugar detox should work fine for you.

How will going on the sugar detox diet help you to lose weight?

Remember earlier in the book we discussed how glucose was converted into glycogen and then being stored in the body? Well when there is no sugars available for your body to burn as energy, your liver will create sugar by itself! How? It will take the glycogen stored in your body fat and change it back to glucose. This process breaks down the fat in your body and turns it into burnable sugar for energy.

Chapter 4:
Sugar Detox Diet

This is based on the 21 Day Sugar Detox diet. The diet works by following the next four steps diligently in order to get the best results from this detox diet:

1. Remove all simple carbs and sugar from your diet for 21 days in a row.

2. Don't eat any foods from the 'Foods to avoid' list.

3. Only eat foods that are on the 'Good foods' list.

4. If you mess up during your detox start over from day one.

Follow the lists provided of foods to avoid and foods to eat during the detox diet. Make sure that you eat lots of the good foods during the 21 days and keep well away from the bad foods. Being diligent about what you are eating during the detox is going to be the key to making sure that the detoxification goes well in your body. Make sure to drink lots of water during the detox to keep yourself hydrated.

Good Foods

Animal Proteins:

- lamb
- eggs
- bacon
- chicken
- deli and cured meats
- bison
- beef
- sausages
- shellfish, clams, mussels, oysters, and other seafood

- veal

- turkey

- white fish

- wild salmon

- tuna

Vegetables that are not starchy:

- brussel sprouts

- bok choy

- bean sprouts

- bamboo shoots

- artichokes

- all leafy dark greens

- garlic

- fennel

- eggplant

- cucumber

- collards

- Chinese cabbage

- celery

- cauliflower

- carrots
- ginger
- green beans
- radishes
- rhubarb
- shallots/green onions
- spinach
- snow peas
- snap peas
- peppers (all kinds)
- leeks
- lettuce
- mushrooms
- kale
- tomato
- turnips
- zucchini
- watercress
- water chestnuts
- yellow squash

Fruits:

- lemons
- limes

Nuts:

- Brazil nuts
- walnuts
- hazelnuts
- almond flour
- almond meal
- pecans
- macadamias
- peanuts
- cashews
- coconut in all of its unsweetened forms: coconut flour, coconut, dried coconut, coconut sugar is not allowed.

Seeds:

- Chia seeds
- apricot seeds
- cocoa 100% is acceptable

- flax seeds

- hemp seeds

- pumpkin seeds

- sunflower seeds

Fats:

- Saturated fats from animal sources- butter, ghee, duck fat, chicken fat, lamb fat, lard, using grass-fed and organic is best.

- Saturated fats from plants- coconut oil, palm oil, organic and unrefined are the best.

Cooking Oils:

- pork or bacon fat

- beef fat

- butter/ghee

- cocoa butter

- duck fat

- palm oil

Oils for Cold Use:

- Avocado oil
- extra virgin olive oil
- flaxseed oil
- nut oils, macadamia, walnut oil, pecan oil
- rice bran oil

Beverages:

- tea, coffee, green, herbal, white teas
- nut milks- unsweetened almond milk, coconut milk
- water, club soda, mineral water

Miscellaneous Condiments:

All herbs are allowed for premixed blends check for hidden ingredients. All spices are allowed.

Capers, fish sauce, hot sauce, tomato paste, gluten-free mustard, kelp flakes, Japanese edible seaweed.

Homemade: ketchup, mayonnaise, salad dressings.

Make sure hummus is made with cauliflower.

Vanilla bean extract, vanilla, almond extract.

Vinegars- Balsamic, apple cider, white, and distilled

Foods to Avoid

If you come across a food that you are not certain about then leave it out.

Refined Carbohydrates:

- Breads of any kind
- pastas, including couscous
- chips
- cereal, granola
- processed rice cakes, oats, popcorn
- sweet treats like candy, cupcakes, cake, cookies, muffins

Processed Foods:

- cut out all processed foods out of your diet during detox

Starchy Vegetables:

- corn
- yams
- sweet potatoes and regular potatoes

Grains:

- anything made from wheat barley, spelt, rye
- flours made from grains or beans

Legumes:

- beans and soy products

Nuts:

- cashews
- peanuts

Fats and Oils:

- buttery spreads such as "I can't believe it's not butter"
- highly processed unsaturated oils like vegetable oil, sunflower oil, canola oil
- hydrogenated or partly hydrogenated oils
- margarine

Sugars or Sweeteners:

- no sugars are allowed
- no natural sweeteners, naturally derived sweeteners

or artificial sweeteners of any kind are allowed.

- No coconut sugar-free
- products that say "sugar free" or artificially sweetened

Drinks:

- alcohol
- juice and other sweet tasting drinks
- milk and dairy
- protein powders that have more than one ingredient
- sodas, including diet sodas

Condiments:

Hummus made from chickpeas or beans, soy sauce, store bought ketchup, mayonnaise, and salad dressings

If you want to do a shorter detox you can try the 3Day Sugar Detox that you follow the basic rules of no fruit (other than lime and lemons), no starches, no wheat, no dairy, and no added sugars. This is a simple kind of cold turkey way to help you to cut your strings to your sugar addiction. Just by doing the 3 Day Sugar Detox you can reverse the signs of premature aging and weight gain caused by sugar. This fast track detox can help you to break free of your sugar addiction immediately. After you have completed the 3 Day Detox you should try and stay on a four-week eating plan with sugar-free recipes.

Once you have completed either the three day or the 21 day detox then use natural sweeteners in very limited quantities. Use natural sweeteners such as:

- cane sugar
- brown sugar
- cane juice crystals
- coconut nectar
- date sugar
- dates
- fruit juice
- honey
- maple syrup
- molasses
- palm sugar
- raw sugar
- Stevia-green leaf or extract

Chapter 5:

Seven Day Sugar Detox Meal Planner

Day 1

Breakfast:

- two hard boiled eggs
- detox smoothie

Lunch:

- Mexican Quinoa Salad

Dinner:

- crumbed cashew chicken

Snack:

- celery sticks and unsweetened peanut butter

Day2

Breakfast:

- detox smoothie
- two poached eggs

Lunch:

- Roasted Brussel sprouts

Dinner:

- Beef Stew

Snack:

- avocado dip with celery sticks

Day3

Breakfast:

- Nutty granola

Lunch:

- Carrot soup

Dinner:

- Slow cooker ham and beans

Snack:

- Oven baked kale chips and avocado dip

Day 4

Breakfast:

- Detox smoothie

Lunch:

- Broccoli Frittata

Dinner:

- Cauliflower soup and apple cider coleslaw

Snack:

- couple of carrot sticks and hummus

Day 5

Breakfast:

- omelet roll

Lunch:

- chicken salad

Dinner:

- tuna fish cakes with pumpkin and eggplant wedges

Snack:

- curry roasted cashews

Day 6

Breakfast:

- spinach smoothie

Lunch:

- egg and bacon ramekins

Dinner:

- Grilled Salmon and asparagus rocket salad

Snack:

- natural nut mix

Day 7

Breakfast:

- scrambled eggs, bacon, tomato, and mushrooms

Lunch:

- kale and radishes, red onion, cucumber salad with homemade balsamic dressing

Dinner:

- Lemon Grass Beef Skewers

Snack:

- pistachios, and cucumber slices with unsweetened peanut butter

Chapter 6:

Sugar Detox Recipes

1. Sugar Detox Smoothie Recipe:

Ingredients:

- squeeze of lemon juice
- one quarter of a cup of cucumber, peeled, seeded
- one cup of unsweetened coconut water
- one cup of kale leaf, chopped
- two sticks of celery, chopped

- one quarter cup of parsley, chopped

- one quarter cup of fresh mint, chopped

- one quarter teaspoon of ginger, grated

Directions:

Place the liquids and other ingredients into a blender and blend well.

2. Mexican Quinoa Salad Recipe:

Ingredients:

- olive oil and vinegar to taste
- basil for garnish
- sea salt to taste
- four tomatoes
- one handful of baby spinach leaves, chopped
- one can of beans
- one cup of quinoa

Directions:

Cook the quinoa according to package instructions. Rinse beans, dice tomatoes, let quinoa cool down add veggies and sprinkle with olive oil, vinegar and salt. Serve chilled.

3. Cashew Crumbed Chicken

Ingredients:

- fourteen ounces of chicken breast cut into thin fillets
- one red onion peeled, finely chopped
- one pinch of sea salt
- handful of crushed cashews or sesame seeds
- three tablespoons of cashew nut meal flour (cashew & almond meal)
- two teaspoons of ground black peppercorns
- two teaspoons of black mustard seeds
- two teaspoons of cumin
- olive oil as needed
- handful of fresh coriander, or parsley, or chives

Directions:

Using a mortar and pestle ground mustard seed and peppercorns. Combine ground pepper, mustard, coriander, cumin and salt in a bowl. Add cashew flour. Heat a pan over medium heat. Add a small amount of oil to pan. Saute onions for five minutes. Remove to a dish.

Add enough oil in the pan to shallow fry chicken which has been coated with cashew and spice mix. Fry chicken till crisp and golden. Return onions for two minutes add seasoning. Serve with a green garden salad. For dressing use a bit of oil with lemon.

4. Roasted Brussels Sprouts

Ingredients:

- two cups of Brussels sprouts
- half a red onion, chopped
- one teaspoon of garlic, minced
- one tablespoon of olive oil
- sea salt to taste

Directions:

Preheat oven to 375 degrees Fahrenheit. Toss all ingredients in a large mixing bowl. Line a baking sheet with parchment paper and place a single layer of Brussels sprouts on it. Roast Brussels sprouts for 30 minutes or until they become golden brown.

5. Beef Stew

Ingredients:

- one pound of cubed beef stew
- two cups homemade beef stock or water
- one small yam, peeled, and cubed
- two carrots, sliced
- two stalks of celery, chopped
- one yellow onion, chopped
- half a red bell pepper, sliced
- one tablespoon of coconut oil
- half a teaspoon of rosemary, dried
- half a teaspoon of parsley, fresh, chopped
- sea salt and black pepper to taste
- add half a cup of tomato or mushrooms if you desire

Directions:

In a large pot cook beef in oil over medium heat until it is browned on all sides. Stir in the rosemary, parsley, salt and pepper. Add beef stock or water, when it starts to boil add yam, carrots, celery, pepper and onion. Cover and cook for another 30 minutes.

6. Avocado Dip

Ingredients:

- two ripe avocados
- two tomatoes
- half a teaspoon of garlic, minced
- half a cup of coriander, fresh, finely chopped or cilantro, finely chopped
- one tablespoon of lime juice
- salt and pepper to taste

Directions:

Make sure that the avocados are nice and ripe. Cut them in half and remove seed and put the pulp into a bowl. Blanche tomatoes, put into boiling water for a few minutes, remove peel. Put all the ingredients into a bowl and mash with a fork. Chill then serve.

7. Nutty Granola

Ingredients:

- three cups of assorted nuts
- two teaspoons of Chia seeds
- one teaspoon of Goji berries
- one tablespoon of sunflower seeds
- two cups of unsweetened coconut, shredded
- half a cup of coconut oil
- one teaspoon of cinnamon
- one quarter cup of sesame seeds

Directions:

Line a baking tray with baking paper and set aside.
Combine the nuts and seeds in a large bowl remove one
cup of nuts and chop into small pieces. Pulse the
remaining seeds and nuts in a blender until they are finely
chopped. Return to mixing bowl with berries and
coconut. Stir well. Place small sauce pan on low heat and
melt oil. Pour hot oil mixture over nut mixture stir and
combine well. Add cinnamon. Pour into baking dish and

press using wet hands. Making sure to pack ingredients well together. Leave mixture for two hours and cover then put into the freezer for at least one hour. Remove from freezer and cut with sharp knife into bars.

8. Raw Carrot Soup

Ingredients:

- two small carrots
- half a cup of cauliflower, florets
- one tomato
- water
- sea salt and black pepper to taste
- ginger, fresh grated to taste
- squeeze of fresh lemon
- half of an avocado

Directions:

Chop up the carrots, tomato, avocado, and cauliflower into chunky pieces, then put them into food processor and blend until smooth. Add water to the amount of how thick you want your soup.

9. Slow Cooker Ham & Beans

Ingredients:

- half a pound of beans of your choice, drained, and rinse.

- One quarter of a pound of cooked ham, chopped

- one teaspoon of onion powder

- water to cover

- sea salt to taste

- pinch of garlic salt and cayenne pepper

Directions:

This can be done on the stove top on simmer for two hours if you do not have a crockpot. In crockpot place all ingredients in on slow cook setting. Pour enough water in it to cover. Set the slow cooker to low and simmer for seven to twelve hours.

10. Oven-baked Kale Chips

Ingredients:

- medium sized bunch of kale
- one quarter teaspoon of sea salt
- three tablespoons of olive oil

Directions:

Wash the kale and remove the hard pieces or stems, tear into bite sized pieces. Sprinkle leaves with salt and olive oil. Toss the kale with fingers to make sure that it is well coated. Bake for ten minutes on a baking sheet at 350 degrees Fahrenheit. Once kale is done place in a bowl and serve immediately after it has cooled.

11. Broccoli Frittata

Ingredients:

- one cup of broccoli, chopped
- four eggs
- half a cup of Tofu
- half a red onion, diced
- one quarter of red bell pepper, chopped
- one teaspoon of organic butter
- one tablespoon of coconut oil
- half a teaspoon of dill, dried
- one quarter teaspoon of sea salt

Directions:

Prepare your tofu according to the directions on package. Mix well until creamy. Mix eggs with the tofu and set aside. Heat the oil and butter in frying pan over medium heat. Once butter has melted saute onions, broccoli, and bell pepper until soft. Add the dill shortly before done. Set vegetables aside. Add egg mixture to the pan turning pan heat to low cover the pan and cook for ten minutes until well done. Serve hot and enjoy!

12. Cauliflower Soup

Ingredients:

- six cups of water
- one small yellow onion, chopped
- one head of cauliflower
- two tablespoons of coconut oil
- sea salt and black pepper to taste
- chopped spring onion, and parsley for garnish

Directions:

Cut the cauliflower into small pieces removing stems and leaves. Fry the onion in saucepan in coconut oil over medium heat for a few minutes. Add the cauliflower and half of water and bring to a simmer. Cover and cook for 15 minutes. Puree the soup in a food processor until it is creamy. Transfer to pot, add salt and pepper, and add more water if you wish to thin the soup. Simmer then serve in serving bowls warm. Garnish with chopped green onion, and parsley.

13. Hummus

Ingredients:

- one 15 ounce can of chickpeas
- one quarter of a cup of tahini
- one large lemon, one quarter cup of lemon juice
- half a teaspoon of garlic, minced
- paprika, for garnish
- two tablespoons of water
- half a teaspoon of ground cumin
- two tablespoons of olive oil

Directions:

In a food processor mix tahini and lemon juice on high. Scrape down sides, add garlic, cumin, salt, and water. Whip for another half minute. Serve with celery sticks or carrot sticks.

14. Omelet Roll

Ingredients:

- one spring onion, thinly sliced
- three eggs
- four tablespoons of cooked lean ham or bacon finely chopped
- sea salt and black pepper to taste
- one tablespoon of coconut oil
- half a cup of mushrooms, sliced
- one tablespoon of milk

Directions:

In a bowl whisk together eggs, milk, salt, pepper, mixing well. Then add the ham, and red pepper and onion. Heat a tablespoon of coconut oil in pan over medium heat. Pour the egg mixture into pan. Fry for a few minutes on both sides, roll up just before serving.

15. Chicken Salad

Ingredients:

- one 15 ounce can of chickpeas, rinsed, and drained
- half a cup of grape tomatoes
- two cups of baby spinach mix
- one cup of cooked chicken, thinly sliced or shaved
- two teaspoons of pumpkin seeds
- use olive oil and lemon juice to make a dressing

Directions:

Combine the tomatoes and chickpeas, along with spinach, chicken other ingredients in a bowl, lightly toss. Serve topped with a lemon olive oil dressing toss lightly again after adding dressing.

16. Tuna Fish Cakes

Ingredients:

- one can of tuna or salmon, drained
- two tablespoons of almond meal
- one cup of shredded zucchini
- one raw egg
- one cup of spring onion, diced
- one quarter teaspoon of sea salt
- half a teaspoon of garlic, minced
- ground black pepper to taste

Directions:

Squeeze out the excess water from zucchini using a paper towel. Add to bowl along with all other ingredients and mix thoroughly. Heat pan and spray with non-stick cooking spray over medium heat. Make small round patties out of mixture and place into the pan. Cook until golden brown on both sides. Serve with pumpkin and eggplant wedges.

17. Curry Roasted Cashews

Ingredients:

- two cups of raw cashews or other nuts such as macadamias
- half a teaspoon of sea salt
- one tablespoon of organic butter
- one quarter teaspoon of ground paprika
- one quarter of a teaspoon of cayenne pepper
- half a teaspoon of natural curry powder
- half a teaspoon of cumin, ground
- half a teaspoon of turmeric, ground
- half a teaspoon of coriander, ground

Directions:

Place all of your spices, cashews, and salt into a bowl and mix well. Spread melted butter across baking pan, preheat oven to 350 degrees Fahrenheit. Place the mixture on top of pan mixing will into the butter. Bake for ten minutes, toss, and bake for another few minutes.

18. Bacon & Egg Ramekins

Ingredients & Directions:

Simply line muffin trays or ramekins with bacon, crack an egg into them at 350 degrees Fahrenheit for ten minutes.

19. Grilled Salmon

Ingredients:

- one pound of salmon fillets
- one medium lemon, sliced
- one teaspoon of coconut oil, melted
- sea salt and black pepper to taste
- dill, fresh, chopped for garnish

Directions:

Put the salmon fillets skin down on a baking sheet that is lined with foil. Season with salt and pepper, place the slices of lemon over salmon. Drizzle lightly with coconut oil. Cover with plastic cling wrap and put in fridge for two hours. Bake in oven at 400 degrees Fahrenheit for 15 minutes.

20. Asparagus Rocket Salad

Ingredients:

- two cups of arugula or rocket mix leafy greens
- salt and pepper to taste
- one tablespoon of apple cider vinegar
- two tablespoons of olive oil
- half a cup of asparagus, chopped
- one cup of tomatoes cut in big pieces
- half a cup of cooked bacon, chopped into small bits

Directions:

In a bowl mix asparagus, tomatoes, and green leaves. In another small bowl mix oil, apple cider vinegar and salt and pepper and add to salad, toss lightly to coat. In serving bowls top with sprinkle of bacon bits and enjoy!

21. Lemon Grass Beef Skewers

Ingredients:

- one pound of lean tenderloin beef cut into small cubes (about half an inch)
- half a teaspoon of garlic, minced
- four stalks of lemon grass
- use anchovies to get a natural fish sauce
- two tablespoons of sesame oil
- two tablespoons of unsweetened coconut water
- one and a half teaspoons of five spice powder
- one small bunch of coriander, chopped

Directions:

Soak your wooden skewers in water for about an hour to prevent them burning. Cut the tops and bottoms away from your lemon grass. Chop remainder of lemon grass finely. Mix with garlic, fish sauce, sesame oil, coconut water, five spice powder, and coriander in a bowl. Marinate your beef cubes in the lemon grass mix for at least 20 minutes. Thread your skewers and fry in oil on stove or on top of BBQ grill. Serve with steamed veggies such as cauliflower or broccoli.

Conclusion

I hope that you will enjoy your experience when you do your sugar detox, hopefully you will find the information suitable in this book that will help you through this process. Just think of how good it will feel when you get rid of the sugar toxins in your body and are able to start a new healthy lifestyle from a fresh start after detoxification. The seven day meal planner and recipes I hope will help to ease your transition a bit by having them to help guide you towards a better healthier version of yourself!

I would also suggest making a specific start date for your sugar detox, add this to your personal calendar. It will allow you time to get yourself psyched to start your sugar detox. It also makes it seem more real when you see it in print. This will give you time to get supplies that you will need during the sugar detox etc. I wish you great success in your sugar detox, you will only gain good from this experience at least from a health perspective—your body will thank you for it I am sure by making you feel the best you have felt in years!

I would like to thank you once again for downloading my book and also ask a small favor in that you leave a small review for the book on Amazon.ca or Amazon.com. It really does help me a lot in improving my books by using the advice given in the reviews. It would be most appreciated if you could take a few moments to leave a quick review—good luck with your sugar detox!

Book 4
The Clean Eating Diet:
Over 30 Delicious and Healthy Clean Eating Recipes To Lose Weight, and Increase Energy Forever!

Introduction

For those living really unhealthy and inactive lifestyles, hearing about the concept of clean eating is like being given a death sentence. They treat this as a scare tactic to get them to move their bodies, start exercising and decreasing their total daily food intake. But in reality, cleaning eating should be that right kind of motivation for them to embark on a quest of finding and rediscovering their best selves.

The Clean Eating Cookbook is the perfect ally that you should have to make sure that you will be able to properly take on the challenge of giving your pantry, grocery list, your cooking and your food choices complete makeovers. How? Well, the book offers you tons of helpful bits of information, which can be very beneficial in ensuring that you will not only lose the weight that you have been trying to shed for many years, at the same time, you and your family will feel more energetic and will soon achieve the best state of health. The book offers:

- Over 30 delicious and really healthy recipes that could jumpstart your weight loss project. From appetizers all the way to your favorite desserts, this book has got your back covered.

- Top tips, including best clean eating practices that you and your family should know and live by. This includes how to start following a clean and healthy lifestyle and the ways to deal and possibly avoid the road blocks that you may or may not encounter.

- Detailed awareness of what clean eating is all about, the different principles that you should learn and practice by heart especially if you are seriously considering turning a new and a healthier "leaf" this year.

- The right kind of encouragement to start buying, cooking and of course, eating healthier and cleaner types of food.

The book aims to help those who needs just the right push to go for their dreams becoming healthier, more energetic and most of all, achieving their optimum health.

Chapter 1: What is Clean Eating

Sometimes, all you need to do is to backtrack your life and think about your eating habits back when your life was a lot simpler. People who have jumped from one weight loss regimen to another are there to attest that for these diets to work, you need to start cleaning up your eating habits. Because amidst the different exercise routines and the diet fads that have gained popularity over the years, once thing is for sure, they all start and end with food!

What is Clean Eating?

The concept of clean eating has been practiced ever since the first man learned how to make use of the natural vegetation and wild animal resources in their areas. It is simply eating organic, lean and naturally obtained fruits, vegetables and meat using the simplest and the healthiest preparations.

Contrary to what most people believe, this practice is not a diet. But rather, clean eating is a lifestyle. This is not something that you can follow just to lose weight and forego once you have achieved your weight loss goals. Eating clean is a practice that you and your family should ultimately live by for the rest of your lives.

To better understand what this healthy lifestyle is all about, you definitely need to find out more about its principles.

The Principles of Clean Eating

Clean eating involves specific principles that does not just cover choosing the healthiest of fruits, vegetables and cuts of meat. It also requires the ability to completely avoid the consumption of certain types of food in order for this new found love for health to work.

- **Cook your own food** – meals prepared at home are known and proven to be several times healthier than your favorite fast food meals. No matter how much these restaurants claim that they use nothing but the best products, you can never be too sure that they do not use processed food products. Clean eating will help you learn how to prepare fast, simple and healthy meals.

- **Consume Whole Foods** – these are food items that have not been altered or laced with fertilizers and other growth inducing chemicals. Think about the concept of "Farm to Table Meals" and you will understand that this is about choosing completely organic and farm raised products.

- **No to Processed Foods** – canned, packed and labeled foods are considered to be processed types of food. The thing about such types of foods is that they may contain ingredients, such as preservatives that could be chemically laced and are harmful to your body. But if there are processed foods that you can eat, those would be whole grain pastas, vegan meat substitutes, organic grains and flours and cheeses. Every time you read the labels, keep in mind that if you cannot pronounce it, do not buy it!

- **Eat Five or Six Meals Everyday** – now this should be done in moderation, to make sure that your body will have enough fuel to burn. These meals should be small and should ultimately be healthy.

- **Having the Right Combination of Carbs and Protein** – this will encourage you to go for more balanced meals every single day. Whether you are snacking or having lunch, your plate should have the right proportions of carbs and protein. This will not only make your healthier, you will also be able to quell all your bouts of hunger and unrealistic cravings.

- **Say No to Refined Sugar** – these are chemically produced, which means that they are harmful and can cause your blood sugar level to dangerously increase.

Through these principles, you will be able to create a more solid and healthy eating habit.

Chapter 2: Benefits of Clean Eating

Now that you know what clean eating is all about, it is time for you to become fully aware of the benefits that you and your family can get out of choosing the types of food you eat and the way you consume food, in general. So what can clean eating do to your body and your overall health?

- **Helps regulates your digestive system's processes** – have you noticed that after eating that large serving of cheese burger and a handful of fries, your stomach feels so full and totally acidic?

Well, if you observe carefully, you will even hear your digestive enzymes struggle to work their way through all the oily processed foods that you have consumed. Clean eating will help put a stop to acid refluxes, indigestion and poor bowel movement. You will have all the fiber that you need to improve your digestion in so many ways.

- **Helps keep you satisfied for longer periods of time** – junk food makes you crave more food, which in turn makes you gain those unwanted pounds. Eating cleaner and healthier food will make sure that you will feel full and satisfied longer since you will be completely nourished.

- **Helps you stay active and energized** – foods that are high in cholesterol can slow you down, not to mention that they can cause serious health problems. But with whole foods, you will be able to not only decrease your cholesterol levels, you will also have enough energy to go through your day from start to finish.

- **Helps keep your body nourished and healthy** – at the end of the day, your main goal is to be healthy, so following a clean eating lifestyle will help you achieve that, plus more. The body will have the energy and the capacity to breakdown your food, enough to extract the right amounts of nutrients and micronutrients to satiate your body's needs to achieve your optimum health. These foods will help lower your cholesterol levels, regulate your sugar intake and strengthen your immune system.

- **Helps you become adventurous and experimental in cooking** – this lifestyle does not mean that you have to eat bland and dull looking meals every single time. Clean eating, with all the amazingly healthy ingredients that you can choose from, should and will encourage you to try new recipes to bring life to your dishes. Clean eating should get you excited to prepare your own meals!

- **Clean eating is for the benefit of everyone**– gone are the days when you think that healthy or clean eating is just for vegans, vegetarians, diabetes, heart patients or those who are on a really strict diet. Clean eating is for those who would like to take great care of themselves better.

Chapter 3:

Clean Eating Lifestyle Tips to Follow When Preparing Your Food

Clean eating can sometimes be discouraging even for those who already know their way around the kitchen. For those who are just starting out, these tips can surely supersize your excitement to prepare your very own healthier versions of your favorite recipes, more so, to try new ones.

- **Spice Up Your Meals** – if you are a bit scared to try new spices and seasoning blends, why don't you go for herbs and other ingredients that could elevate and take your healthy meals to whole new levels? Try experimenting and incorporating these healthy herbs and spices in your next recipes:

- Cloves

- Cinnamon

- Nutmeg

- Cumin

- Turmeric

- Sage

- Mint

- Rosemary

- Basil

- Marjoram

- o Chili

- o Thyme

- **Plan your meals** – there are several ways to diversify your meals on a daily basis. Make the internet your best friend, or this book to look for amazingly delicious but unbelievably healthy dishes that you can easily make for your family. You can create a chart and plan what you will be cooking and eating for a week or in the next few days.

- **Experiment in the kitchen** – do not be afraid to get out of your comfort zone and experiment on different healthy recipes that you have found. You can try small portions first and see if you and the rest of the family will like what you have prepared.

- **Cook your meals ahead** – you really do not have to be a slave in the kitchen every day, because there are healthy or nutritious meals that you can make ahead of time, store in the fridge and reheat. You can even label the containers with the dates or day that they should be consumed to keep their freshness and maintain their flavors.

- **Make a list** – do not get too overly excited to shop for fruits, veggies, meats and dairy products. Keep a record of what ingredients you have and take note of their expiration dates; this list will serve are your reference for the next time that you will go grocery shopping.

With all these in mind, it is definitely time to start cooking!

Chapter 4: 30 Amazing Recipes to Improve Your Health

Starting from your appetizers, you will now have the chance to really try following a healthier and cleaner lifestyle.

Healthy Appetizers You Should Try Making

Set the right tone for healthy eating by making these easy appetizer recipes:

Mozzarella, Basil and Tomato Skewers

Ingredients:

- 16 pieces of fresh buffalo mozzarella balls

- 16 pieces of cherry tomatoes

- 16 pieces of fresh basil leaves

- Olive oil

- Sea salt and freshly cracked black pepper

- Small skewers

Instructions

- Take a small skewer and thread a piece of mozzarella ball, a piece of basil leaf and a cherry tomato. Do this process until you have made 16 skewers and drizzle with olive oil. Season with salt and pepper.

- Amp up the flavors by lightly grilling them.

Balsamic Tomato Bruschetta

Ingredients:

- 8 plum or Roma tomatoes de-seeded and diced

- 1/3 cup of basil chopped

- ¼ of parmesan cheese shredded

- 2 large garlic cloves minced

- 1 Tablespoons of high quality balsamic vinegar

- 1 teaspoon of olive oil

- ¼ teaspoon of sea or kosher salt

- ¼ teaspoon of black pepper

- 1 loaf of French bread sliced and toasted.

Instructions

- In a large bowl combine tomatoes, cheese, basil and garlic together. Add in the balsamic vinegar, olive oil, salt and pepper. Cover and let the mixture marinate in the fridge for at least 30 minutes to let the flavors marry together.

- Once ready to serve, toast the slices of French bread drizzled in olive oil. Spoon the marinated tomato mixture and serve.

Lemon and Thyme Ricotta Dip

Ingredients:

- 1 15 ounce container of fresh, part skim ricotta cheese

- 2 tablespoons of fresh thyme chopped

- 2 tablespoons of shallot, minced or chopped finely

- 1 teaspoon of fresh chives, chopped

- 2 teaspoons of lemon zest

- ¼ cup of freshly squeezed lemon juice

- ½ teaspoon of sea salt

- 1 teaspoon of black or white pepper

- 2 teaspoons of extra virgin olive oil

Instructions

- Using a blender, food processor or regular mixer, whip together the ricotta, thyme, chives, shallots, lemon zest and juice, salt and pepper until light and smooth.

- Place in a bowl and drizzle with 2 teaspoons of olive oil. Serve with fresh vegetables, wheat thins, naan or tortilla chips.

Easy Homemade Kale Chips

Ingredients:

- 1 large bunch of fresh kale

- 1 Tablespoon of olive oil

- 1 tablespoon of sherry vinegar

- 1/8 teaspoons of kosher or sea salt

Instructions

- Preheat your oven to 150 degrees Centigrade.

- Trim and prep your kale by taking the ribs out of each leaf. Dry the kale and drizzle with olive oil. Toss the leaves by hand to ensure that each is coated with oil. Sprinkle with vinegar and toss well.

- Line a baking sheet with a silicone baking sheet or parchment paper and evenly spread the leaves.

- Bake for about 35 minutes or until the chips are crispy.

- Season with salt and serve as is or with some homemade tartar sauce.

Goat Cheese Stuffed Tomatoes

Ingredients

- 24 pieces of cherry tomatoes

- 3 ounces of fresh goat cheese

- 1 tablespoon of low fat milk

- 2 tablespoons of chopped green or black olives

- 2 teaspoons of chopped oregano (fresh)

- 1/8 teaspoons of pepper

Instructions

- Slice the tops of each cherry tomato and scoop out the seeds (if any). Set aside and start preparing the filling.

- Mix the goat cheese, olives, milk, pepper and oregano together to form a paste.

- Fill each tomato's cavity and drizzle with olive oil, more oregano and pepper. You can chill these before serving.

Healthy Black Bean Salsa

Ingredients

- 3 cans or about 3 and ½ cups of black beans. You can buy dried ones and cook them until tender

- 1 cup of Mexican corn or 1 can of corn

- 4 large fresh Roma tomatoes, diced

- 1 large green chili pepper (Jalapeno)

- ½ cup of green onions, chopped

- 1 bunch of cilantro leaves

- Salt and pepper to taste

Instructions

- Mix together all the ingredients, except for the cilantro leaves. If you want the cilantro taste to come together with the rest of the mixture, you may chop half of the bunch and toss it in. Season with salt and pepper.

- Place the mixture in a bowl, top with the remaining cilantro leaves and serve with tortilla, corn chips or crackers.

Crispy Polenta Wedges with Tomato Tapenade

Ingredients

- 1 tube of pre-made polenta (you can make your own by cooking polenta on a stove, according to package direction and spread onto a lined baking sheet and chill to solidify.)

- Cooking spray or canola oil

- 2/3 cup of sun dried tomatoes (canned or jarred)

- 4 teaspoons of olive oil

- 1 tablespoon of chopped flat-leaf parsley

- 2 teaspoons of capers, rinsed to remove the excess salt

- 1 garlic clove minced

- 1/8 teaspoons of pepper

Instructions

- Preheat your oven to 350 degrees and line a baking sheet with parchment paper and spray some non-stick cooking spray over the paper. You can also oil the sheet with canola oil.

- Slice the polenta into wedges or triangles and place them, evenly spaced, onto the baking pan. Bake the polenta wedges for about 15 minutes or until the edges are crispy and let them cool.

- In a food processor, blend the tomatoes parsley, garlic, olive oil, capers and pepper into a thick but not so smooth paste.

- Top each polenta wedge with the tomato tapenade, sprinkle parsley and serve.

Quick and Easy Hummus

Ingredients

- 1 can or about 15 ounces of cooked garbanzo beans or chick peas

- 2 ounces of fresh Jalapeno peppers, sliced into rounds

- ½ teaspoon of cumin (powder)

- 2 Tablespoons of lemon juice

- 3 large cloves of garlic, chopped

Instructions

- Using a food processor, combine all ingredients together to form a paste. If the mixture is too thick, add a little bit of the chickpea water. Keep adding until you have reached the desired consistency.

- Place the hummus in a bowl and serve with sliced flat bread, pita chips or paratha.

Thai-Style Chicken Balls

Ingredients

- 2 lbs. of minced chicken

- 1 cup bread crumbs

- 4 green onions, chopped

- 1 tablespoons of coriander powder

- 1 cup of fresh cilantro, chopped

- ¼ cup of Thai sweet chili sauce

- 2 tablespoons of freshly squeezed lemon juice

- Canola oil for frying

Instructions

- In a bowl, mix together chicken, bread crumbs, chopped green onions, coriander powder, cilantro, chili sauce and lemon juice together. Form balls out of the mixture and set aside. Chill the prepared chicken balls to make sure that it is firm enough for frying.

- Meanwhile, heat oil in a deep pot or fryer. Once the chicken balls are firm enough, fry each ball in hot oil.

Steak and Blue Cheese Wrapped Bell Peppers

Ingredients

- 16 thinly sliced steak, grilled

- 1 cup of blue cheese or goat's cheese

- 4 large red and yellow bell peppers cut into strips.

Instructions

- Spread a generous amount of cheese onto each steak.

- Place about 3 or 4 pepper strips on top of the cheese and roll each piece of steak to form a log. Secure each with a toothpick.

Entrees or Main Courses

Breakfast, lunch or dinner, the main course will always be the meal that will convince you and your family that healthy and clean eating is definitely the way to go.

Quick Tomato-Mozzarella Pizza

Ingredients

- 1 frozen whole wheat pizza dough (you can also use large tortillas or flat breads)

- 2 tablespoons of yellow cornmeal or course corn flour

- 5 large plum tomatoes, sliced thinly

- 1 large clove of garlic, minced

- 1 cup of shredded fresh mozzarella cheese

- ¼ teaspoons of black pepper

- ¼ cup of basil, sliced into thin strips

*you can also use bacon or pancetta slices

Instructions

- Preheat your oven to 350 degrees. If you have a pizza stone, you may place the stone in the oven to heat up.

- Prepare the dough by sprinkling some cornmeal all over the edges. Sprinkle the rest of the cornmeal onto a baking sheet or your pizza stone.

- Spread the minced garlic all over the dough and sprinkle half of the cheese on top. Arrange the tomatoes on top and sprinkle the basil leaves.

- Add the rest of the cheese and bake for about 10 minutes or until the cheese has melted. Slice and serve.

Vegetarian Burgers

Ingredients

- 1 medium sized zucchini, grated

- 1 potato, grated

- 1 medium carrot, grated

- ¼ cup of onions, minced

- ½ teaspoon of chopped oregano

- 2 egg whites or egg replacer equivalent to 2 eggs

Instructions

- Mix all the ingredients together. Make sure that everything has been incorporated well.

- Form into patties in your desired size and thickness and place in the chiller to firm up.

- Heat a pan with a little bit of cooking oil and fry each patty when firm.

Quick Baked Halibut

Ingredients

- 1 teaspoon of olive oil

- 1 cup medium zucchini, diced

- ½ cup of onion, chopped

- 1 large clove of garlic, grated

- 2 cups of Roma tomatoes, diced

- 2 tablespoons of basil, chopped

- ¼ teaspoon of salt

- ¼ teaspoon of ground black pepper

- 2 halibut steaks

- 1/3 cup of feta cheese, crumbled

Instructions

- Preheat your oven to 450 degrees. Line a baking tray with parchment or baking paper.

- In a medium sauce pan, heat olive oil and sauté the garlic, onions and zucchini. Once the zucchini has soften, turn off the heat and stir in the tomatoes, basil and season with salt and pepper.

- Place the halibut steaks on the baking sheet and top with the sautéed vegetables. Drizzle with a little bit of olive oil and bake for about 15 to 20 minutes.

Cornflake Crusted Chicken with Pineapple Salsa

Ingredients

Salsa

- 1 cup of chopped fresh pineapple

- 2 tablespoons of fresh cilantro leaves, chopped

- 1 tablespoon of finely chopped red onion

- Chicken

- 1/3 cup of lightly crushed plain corn flakes

- 1 cup panko break crumbs or herbed Italian bread crumbs

- ½ teaspoon of salt

- A pinch of pepper

- 4 large chicken cutlets or chicken breast fillet (skinless)

- 1 ½ teaspoons of canola oil for frying, add more if you are using a non-stick pan

Instructions

- Make the salsa first by combing all the ingredients together. Place in an air tight container and refrigerate.

- Combine cornflakes. Salt, pepper and bread crumbs in a small bowl. You can add other herbs such as cilantro, parsley and even paprika. Coat each cutlet with the cornflake mixture and set aside.

- Chill the chicken cutlets and heat your pan.

- Fry the chicken pieces until golden brown. You may bake the chicken fillets in a 450 degree oven for about 15-20 minutes. Serve in a platter with some pineapple salsa on the side.

Lean and Healthy Meatloaf

Ingredients

- 1 lb. turkey breast, minced

- 1 lb. of lean beef, minced

- ¼ cup of sun dried tomatoes or about 2 tablespoons of tomato paste

- 1 cup of red onion, diced

- 1 cup bell pepper, finely chopped

- ½ cup of carrot, diced finely

- 1 cup of zucchini, grated

- ¼ cup of chopped parsley

- 2 whole eggs

- ½ teaspoon of fresh thyme

- 4 large cloves of garlic, crushed

- ½ cup of panko bread crumbs

- ¼ cup ground flaxseed

- ¼ teaspoon of pepper, salt

- ¼ cup of organic chicken broth

Instructions

- Preheat your oven to 350 degrees and grease a large loaf pan with baking spray or canola oil. You can line it with parchment paper as well.

- Mix all the ingredients together until well combined.

- Place the mixture in the prepared pan and bake for about 1 ½ to 2 hours. Watch over the meatloaf because it can dry out easily, since you will be using turkey and lean meat. If using meat thermometer, the center of the meatloaf should be within the 150 to about 170 degrees.

- Let the cooked meatloaf rest and cool off a bit before unmolding and slicing.

Szechwan Shrimps

Ingredients

- 12 ounces of medium shrimps – peeled, de-veined and butterflied

- 4 cloves of garlic, chopped

- ¼ cup chopped green onions

- ¼ teaspoon ginger powder

- 1 tablespoon of ground nut oil/ peanut oil

- ½ teaspoon of red pepper flakes

- 2 tablespoons of ketchup

- 4 tablespoons of water

- 1 tablespoon of tamari or light soy sauce

- 1 teaspoon of honey or agave

- 2 teaspoons of cornstarch

Instructions

- Prepare the sauce by mixing all the wet ingredients together. Add in the red pepper flakes, cornstarch and ground ginger and stir well.

- In a large wok, heat oil and sauté the garlic and green onions until fragrant. Add the shrimps and cook until they are almost cooked and immediately stir in the sauce mixture.

- Wait until the shrimps are fully cooked and the sauce has thickened before turning off the heat. Serve with cooked brown rice.

Cumin and Coriander Crusted Steak

Ingredients

- 1 tablespoon of brown sugar, packed

- 1.2 teaspoon of salt

- ½ teaspoon of pepper

- ½ teaspoon of cumin powder

- ½ teaspoon of coriander powder

- ¼ teaspoon of red pepper powder

- 1 lb. boneless sirloin steak

Instructions

- Preheat your oven to 450 degrees. Coat a thick oven safe pan or cast iron skillet with oil and place it inside the oven to heat up.

- Combine all the ingredients together and rub all over the prepared steak.

- Place the steak in the pan and bake for about 7 minutes for medium cook. Slice thinly, against the grain.

Hawaiian Chicken

Ingredients

- 2 pieces of large chicken breast fillet

- ¼ teaspoon each of the following spices:

    o Ginger

    o Paprika

- ¾ teaspoon of onion powder

- 1 ½ teaspoon of garlic powder

- 1 tablespoon of apple cider vinegar

- ¼ cup of tomato sauce

- 1 tablespoon of soy sauce or tamari

- 1 5 ounce can of crushed pineapple

- ½ tablespoon of brown sugar

- Cooked brown rice

Instructions

- Preheat your oven to about 400 degrees and line a baking sheet with parchment paper.

- Place the chicken fillets in the pan and set aside.

- Mix together the onion, garlic, paprika and ginger powders and add in the vinegar. Baste the top of the chicken with the mixture and bake for about 10 minutes.

- After 10 minutes, turn the chicken and baste the top with the remaining vinegar mixture and place it back in the oven.

- In a small bowl, mix the remaining ingredients together except the brown rice. Coat the chicken fillets with the ketchup and pineapple mixture and bake for another 15 minutes or until the chicken fillets have formed crusts.

- Serve on top of a plate of cooked brown rice.

Healthy Chickpea Curry

Ingredients

- 2 cans or 2 cups of cooked garbanzo beans or chickpeas

- 2 T of vegetable oil

- 2 red onions, chopped

- 2 large cloves of garlic, crushed

- 2 teaspoons of fresh ginger, grated

- 6 whole cloves

- 2 sticks of cinnamon

- 1 teaspoon of ground cumin

- 1 teaspoon of ground coriander

- Salt to taste

- 1 teaspoon of cayenne pepper

- 1 teaspoon of turmeric powder

- 1 cup of chopped cilantro

- ½ cup Vegetable stock

Instructions

- Heat oil in the pan and saute all your aromatics (garlic, onions and ginger) until fragrant. Add in your spices and fry the mixture until you can smell all the spices.

- Stir in the garbanzo beans and saute for about 5 minutes.

- Add the stock and simmer for 10 to 15 minutes. Adjust seasoning to taste. Top with fresh cilantro leaves.

All-Spice Pork Chops with Mango Salsa

Ingredients

- ¾ teaspoon of chili powder

- ¼ teaspoon of sea salt

- 1/8 teaspoon of all spice powder

- 4 medium sized pork chops (de-boned)

- 1 and a half cups of diced mangoes (ripe)

- 2 tablespoons of fresh mint, chopped

- 1 tablespoons of lemon juice (fresh)

- 2 teaspoons of sugar

- ¼ teaspoons of red pepper flakes

Instructions

- Prepare the marinade for the pork. Mix together the all spice powder, salt and chili powder. Evenly coat the pork with the spice blend and chill for about 20 minutes.

- Heat a skillet and add oil. Once the chops are ready, pan fry each chop, about 4 to 5 minutes per side or until cooked evenly.

- While waiting for the pork to cook, prepare your salsa by combining the rest of the ingredients. Chill the mango salsa.

- Place 2 pieces of chops per plate and top with mango salsa to serve.

Tomato and Spinach Angel Hair Pasta

Ingredients

- 1 cup of vegetable stock

- 12 pieces of sundried tomatoes

- 2 tablespoons of toasted pine nuts

- ¼ teaspoon of crushed red pepper flakes

- 1 large clove of garlic, crushed

- 1 bunch of fresh spinach leaves, torn into bite size pieces.

- ¼ cup parmesan cheese, grated

- 8 ounces of angel hair pasta, cooked according to package direction

- Salt and pepper to taste

Instructions

- In a large sauce pan, sauté garlic and red pepper flakes until fragrant. Add in the spinach and sun dried tomatoes and cook until the tomatoes have soften. Pour the broth and simmer for about 4 minutes.

- Add the cooked pasta, toss in the pine nuts and simmer until the pasta has absorbed the sauce. Mix well and serve. Sprinkle with parmesan cheese.

Clean, Healthy and Scrumptious Desserts and Snacks

Healthy and Light Frozen Peanut Butter Yogurt

Ingredients

- 2 cups of plain or vanilla flavored yogurt – none or low fat yogurt works too!

- ½ cup milk (dairy or non-dairy)

- ½ cup peanut butter or any nut butter of your choice

- 1 ½ teaspoon of pure vanilla extract

- ¼ teaspoon of sea salt

- 1/3 cup of natural sugar (agave/maple)

Instructions

- In a food processor or blender, mix together all the ingredients until thoroughly combined.

- Place in individual cups, ramekins or air tight containers and freeze. Top with crushed cacao nibs, crushed peanut butter cups or cookies before serving.

Date and Oatmeal Cookies

Ingredients

- 2 large ripe bananas

- 5 large Medjool pitted dates

- 2 cups of rolled oats – gluten free

- Pinch of cinnamon and sea salt

Instructions

- Preheat your oven to 350 degrees and line a baking pan with parchment or baking paper.

- Using a food processor, blend the oats until it reaches a coarse texture. Add in the dates and blend. Add the bananas and the rest of the ingredients to form a dough.

- Scoop out the dough and make about 1 inch balls. Place them evenly on the prepared tray and bake for about 17 minutes. Let the cookies cool before serving.

Non-Dairy Avocado Ice Cream
Tropicale

Ingredients

- 2 large ripe avocados, pitted and sliced

- 1 can (15 ounces) pineapple bites, reserve the juice

- ½ cup of coconut milk

- 3 Tablespoons Fresh Lime Juice

- A pinch of sea salt

- ½ cup of raw cocoa powder

- ½ coconut oil

- ¼ cup of maple syrup

Instructions

- Spread the avocado and pineapple slices onto a baking sheet and freeze for 3 hours.

- Process the frozen fruits until the mixture forms a smooth paste and then slowly add the lime juice, pineapple juice, coconut milk, salt and vanilla. Place the mixture in an air tight or covered bowl and freeze until needed.

- While waiting for the avocado ice cream to freeze, prepare the chocolate shards or chips.

- Melt the coconut oil (if solid) and add the cocoa powder. Mix well before adding the maple syrup. Pour the mixture in a lined pan and freeze to solidify.

- Run the avocado mixture in your ice cream maker to churn. It may take about 20 minutes.

- Scoop out the ice cream in bowls and garnish with chocolate shards.

No-Bake Healthy Coconut Snow-Balls

Ingredients

- 1 ¾ cups unsweetened coconut shreds, divided plus a little bit of extra

- 2 teaspoons coconut oil, melted

- 3 tablespoons of maple syrup

- ½ teaspoon vanilla

- ½ teaspoon cinnamon powder

- 1/8 teaspoon of salt

Instructions

- In a food processor, blend together 1 cup of the coconut shreds and the coconut oil until the mixture turns into a paste.

- Add the maple syrup, vanilla, cinnamon and salt. Once incorporated, mix in the rest of the coconut shreds. The mixture will be doughy but not firm.

- Form the dough into balls and dredge them in the remaining coconut flakes. Chill for about an hour.

Mango-Colada Popsicles

Ingredients

- 2 cups frozen mango (organic)

- ¾ cup unsweetened coconut milk

- 1 cup unsweetened full fat coconut cream/milk

- 1 and half tablespoons of honey or agave or coconut nectar for vegans

Instructions

- Puree the frozen mango and add about ¼ cup of the unsweetened coconut milk.

- In a small bowl, add the rest of the coconut milk, 1 cup of the canned coconut cream and your chosen sweetener.

- Prepare your Popsicle molds. Pour 2 tablespoons of mango puree into the molds, let it set for a bit and pour the creamy mixture on top. Cover the molds and insert the sticks. Freeze solid.

Raw Brownies

Ingredients

- 1 cup raw pecans or walnuts

- 1 cup Medjool dates, pitted

- 5 tablespoons of raw cacao or raw cocoa powder

- 2 tablespoons of agave nectar, maple syrup or honey

- ¼ teaspoon sea salt

Instructions

- In a food processor, grind the pecans until it becomes coarse, add the dates. As soon as the mixture becomes sticky, it is now ready for the rest of the ingredients.

- Blend the rest of the ingredients and pour the mixture in a lined baking sheet. Spread evenly and refrigerate for at least 3 hours.

Melon and Apple Granita

Ingredients

- 4 cups of ripe melon, cubed

- 1 cup unsweetened apple juice (bottled or fresh)

- ¼ cup fresh lime juice

- 1 cup blueberries (fresh)

- 1 cup raspberries (fresh)

- Mint leaves for garnish

Instructions

- Blend all ingredients together (except the mint leaves) and pour the liquid mixture into a shallow pan.

- Place the pan in the freezer and let the mixture set for about 3 to 4 hours. Take the pan out and scrape the slightly frozen mixture. Place it back in the freezer.

- Do it again after an hour and let it freeze again. Take the granita out 30 minutes before serving. Scoop the granite into cups and garnish with mint leaves.

Healthy Peachy Green Smoothie

Ingredients

- 2 cups of frozen peaches (if using fresh, freeze them first for about 4 hours)

- 2 cups of spinach leaves

- 1 cup of water

- 1 tablespoon of grated fresh ginger

- 1 tablespoon of honey or agave

Instructions

- Pour water, honey, ginger and spinach in a blender and pulse. The mixture should be smooth and really green.

- Add the frozen peaches and blend until it forms a smoothie-like consistency.

- Serve in chilled tall glasses.

Super Healthy Vegan Nutella

Ingredients

- 2 cups of raw hazelnuts

- 1 ½ cups of melted dark chocolate

- 1/3 cup raw coconut sugar

- 1 tablespoon coconut oil

- 1 teaspoons of vanilla extract

- ¾ teaspoon of salt

Instructions

- Blend the raw hazelnuts into a fine paste and add the rest of the ingredients.

- Store the prepared hazelnut spread in a jar and store in the fridge.

Banana Pudding Pots

Ingredients

- 10 pieces of raw almonds- roasted

- 2 tablespoons of cornstarch

- a pinch of salt

- 3 tablespoons of raw coconut or palm sugar

- 1 beaten egg yolk

- ¾ cup of milk (dairy or non-dairy)

- ½ teaspoon of vanilla extract

- 2 ripe bananas, sliced thinly

- 6 dessert cups

Instructions

- In a food processor, grind the almonds and set aside.

- In a small pot, mix together sugar, cornstarch and salt. Add the egg yolk and slowly pour the milk. Heat the mixture until it thickens.

- Remove the pan from the heat and add the vanilla. Let it cool slightly.

- Prepare the cups by placing a layer of the sliced bananas, topped with the custard cream mixture. Create another layer of bananas and cream until the entire cup has been filled. Sprinkle the chopped almonds. You can choose to serve them cold or warm.

Sugar Free Chocolate Covered Strawberries (Paleo)

Ingredients

- ½ kilos of fresh strawberries, cleaned and patted dry

- 1/3 cup of pure cacao powder

- 1 teaspoon of vanilla bean paste

- A pinch of salt and a teaspoon of honey

- 3 tablespoons of coconut oil, melted

Instructions

- Line a baking sheet with parchment paper.

- In a small bowl, combine cocoa powder, vanilla bean paste, melted coconut oil, salt and honey.

- Dip each strawberry into the chocolate mixture and place on the parchment lined pan.

- Chill or let it set in room temperature.

Conclusion

Clean eating is not that difficult to follow, with all these amazing recipes, tips and guidelines, the only thing that you are left to do is to put everything that you have learned here into action. And once you have gotten used to this really simple, healthy and clean lifestyle, you will be able to achieve that energized and fit body that you have always wanted.

This book hopes that you will keep all the principles mentioned here in mind – from choosing to buy unprocessed whole foods, to cutting back on your sugar intake – because at the end of the day, your main goal is not just to lose those extra pounds, but to also influence and encourage others to take on the clean eating lifestyle.

Finally, if you enjoyed this book, then I'd like to ask you for a big favor, would you be kind enough to leave a review for this book on Amazon? It'd be greatly appreciated!

Free Bonus

As my way of saying thank you for reading this book, I've included a very special gift for you; I want to give you a complete e-book called "Weight Loss Enigma".

With this great eBook you'll discover:

- How to lose weight successfully by understanding what the breaking down of food is like within our body...
- Why using food diary could help you to lose weight...
- Identifying your Health and Weight Profile for Successful Weight Loss...
- How to get into shape by exercise that do not required you to visit to the gym?
- Find out the eight most handful tips and effective method in losing weight...
- And much more...

With this special gift you will learn the secret of how to effectively shedding off the excessive bulging belly & stay a healthy shape in no time!

Copy the link below in your browser. My friend

David Smith (who is my publisher) will send you the eBook to your email.

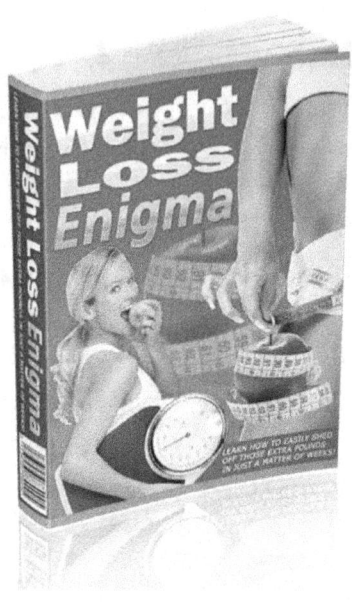

Link:

http://bit.ly/1AhFYqk

DISCLAIMER AND/OR LEGAL NOTICES: Every effort has been made to accurately represent this book and it's potential. Results vary with every individual, and your results may or may not be different from those depicted. No promises, guarantees or warranties, whether stated or implied, have been made that you will produce any specific result from this book. Your efforts are individual and unique, and may vary from those shown. Your success depends on your efforts, background and motivation.

The material in this publication is provided for educational and informational purposes only and is not intended as medical advice. The information contained in this book should not be used to diagnose or treat any illness, metabolic disorder, disease or health problem. Always consult your physician or health care provider before beginning any nutrition or exercise program. Use of the programs, advice, and information contained in this book is at the sole choice and risk of the reader.